ABCs
OF THE
BRACHIAL PLEXUS

WRITTEN BY

DENISE JUSTICE

EDITED BY

HOLLY WAGNER

ILLUSTRATED BY

ALEXANDRA PAQUIN
BETHANY RUNYON

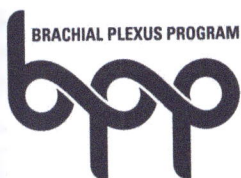

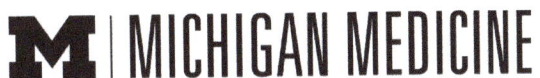

Published in the United States of America by
Michigan Publishing Services
https://services.publishing.umich.edu/
Manufactured in the United States of America

DOI: https://doi.org/10.3998/mpub.11554234

ISBN 978-1-60785-571-2 (paper)
ISBN 978-1-60785-572-9 (e-book)
ISBN 978-1-60785-619-1 (open-access)

This book is dedicated to the patients with neonatal brachial plexus palsy and their families, the medical providers who care for them, and my family who inspires me every single day.

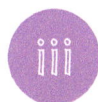

CONTENTS

FOREWORD

The optimal treatment of neonatal brachial plexus palsy (NBPP) requires interdisciplinary collaboration among specialties, such as Neurosurgery/Neurology, Orthopedic Surgery, Hand/Plastic Surgery, and Physiatry. As such, the associated medical terminology and health literacy can be problematic for patients and caregivers.

In this book, Ms. Justice, her co-authors, and illustrators present the most common NBPP medical terminology in a clear, concise, yet visually attractive format that appeals to children and adults alike. The alphabetized and illustrated presentations are supplemented with pithy text to educate the reader in short segments, that either can stand alone or flow into a story of NBPP. This publication not only serves as a valuable resource for patients undergoing treatment for NBPP and their caregivers—but can also serve as a high-yield reference for providers.

The reader will enjoy perusing or studying, in more detail, the included medical vocabulary. Ms. Justice's *ABCs of the Brachial Plexus* is a worthy addition to the published literature.

Lynda J-S Yang, MD, PhD
Director, Brachial Plexus and Peripheral Nerve Program
Professor, Department of Neurosurgery
University of Michigan

ABOUT THE AUTHOR

Denise Justice, OTRL, FMiOTA, is an Occupational Therapist in the interdisciplinary Brachial Plexus Program at the University of Michigan. As a graduate of Eastern Michigan University with a Bachelor of Science degree, Denise later developed a subspecialty interest in the care of children with NBPP. Since 2006, Denise has been particularly dedicated to improving the education of and consequent quality of care for her patients and families, and has authored other publications on this condition. She is actively involved in local, national, and international organizations that foster clinical practice, patient education, and research, with the goal of improving patient outcomes. In 2018, Denise received the "Roster of Fellows" award for her contributions to the profession of Occupational Therapy within the state of Michigan.

ABOUT THE ILLUSTRATORS

Alexandra Paquin is a fine artist with an affinity for depicting the human figure. She studied at Spring Arbor University where she earned a Bachelor of Arts degree with concentrations in both drawing and painting. Her undergraduate studies explored a wide variety of media, though oils have remained her primary focus. This project provided the opportunity to create illustrations that offered both the human figure as a subject and a chance to further explore ink and watercolor, and was a thrilling and challenging venture.

Bethany Runyon graduated from Spring Arbor University with a Bachelor of Arts degree; her concentration was in both drawing and graphic design. She blends her interest in art with a desire to improve the quality of life for those facing medical challenges. Bethany describes her contribution to the illustrations within this book as an honor.

ACKNOWLEDGMENTS

Funding for this project was provided by a generous contribution from MedSAU, supporting a collaborative effort between the Interdisciplinary Brachial Plexus and Peripheral Nerve Program at University of Michigan and Spring Arbor University. Special thanks to the faculty, staff, and regents of the University of Michigan Brachial Plexus / Peripheral Nerve Program, the Neurosurgery Department, and our patients.

ABCs
OF THE
BRACHIAL PLEXUS

IS FOR ADL. ADL STANDS FOR ACTIVITIES OF DAILY LIVING. ACTIVITIES OF DAILY LIVING CAN INCLUDE DRESSING, BATHING, GROOMING, AND SELF-FEEDING. ARM WEAKNESS CAN LEAD TO LIMITATIONS IN COMPLETING THESE AND OTHER DAILY ACTIVITIES.

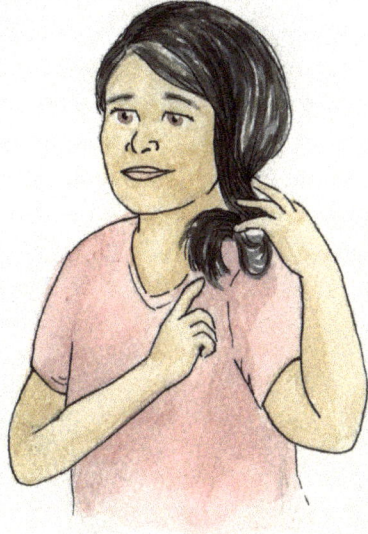

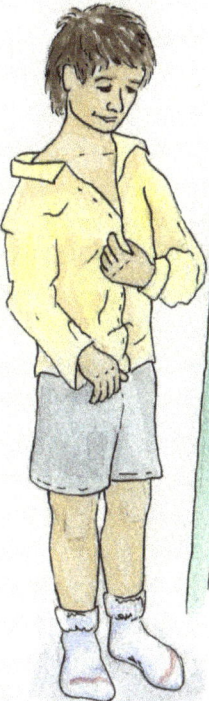

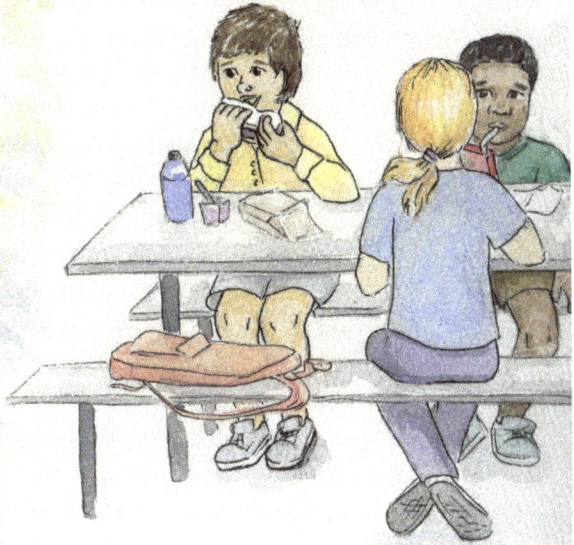

A IS FOR ARM. ARM WEAKNESS HAPPENS WHEN NERVES OF THE BRACHIAL PLEXUS ARE STRETCHED.

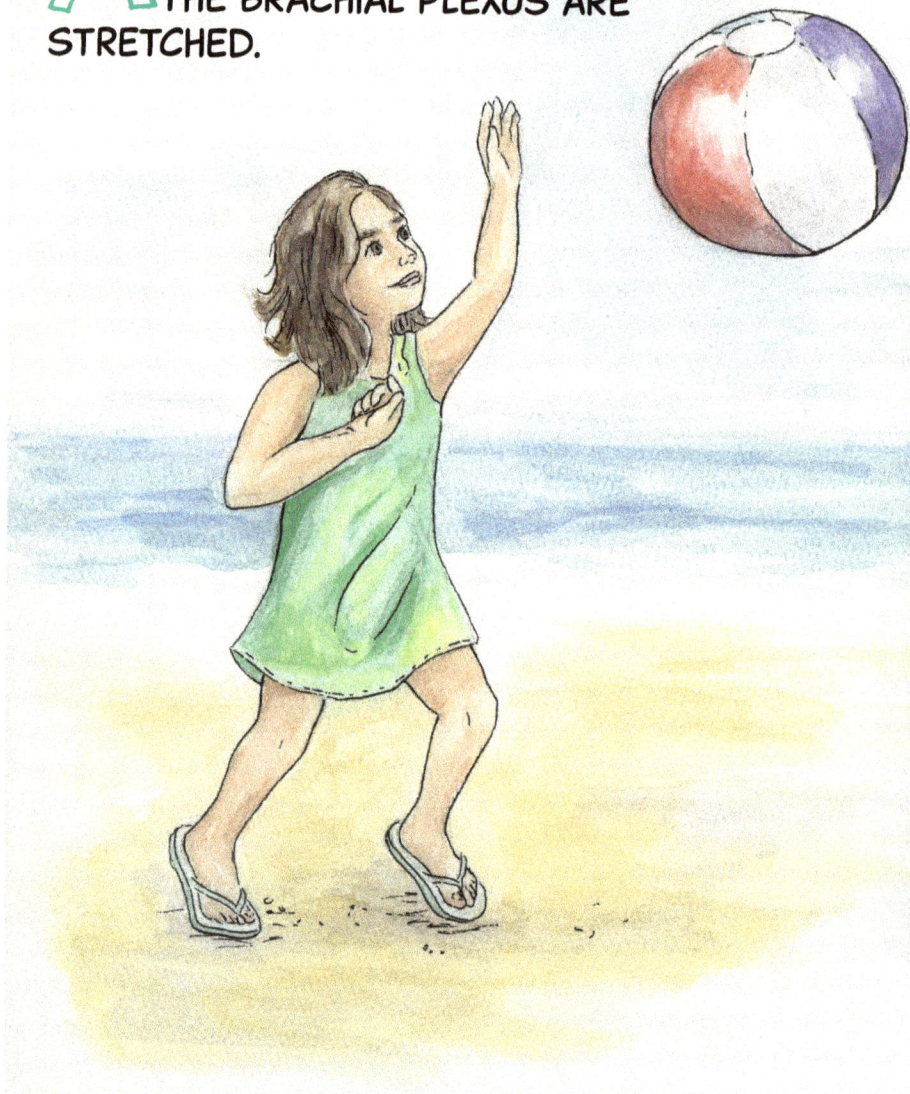

ABCs OF THE BRACHIAL PLEXUS

IS FOR AVULSION.
AVULSION MEANS A
NERVE OF THE BRACHIAL
PLEXUS IS PULLED AWAY FROM
THE SPINAL CORD.

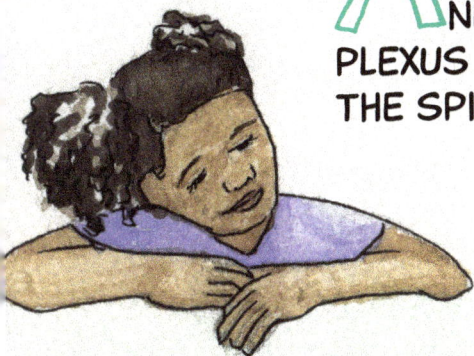

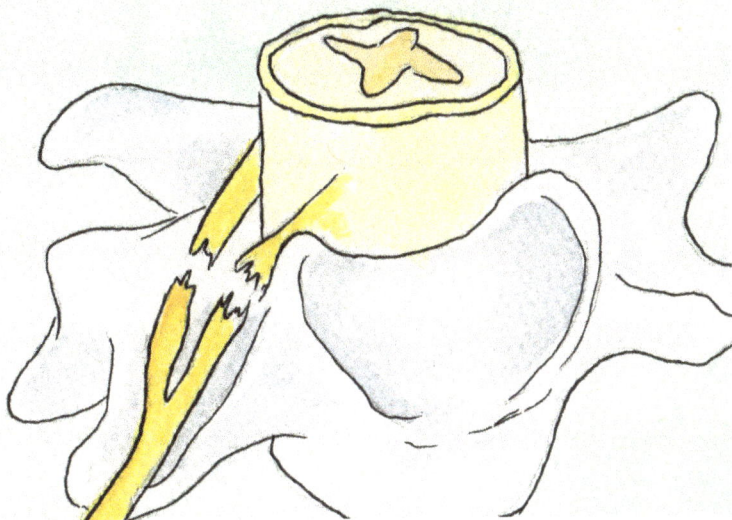

ABCs OF THE BRACHIAL PLEXUS

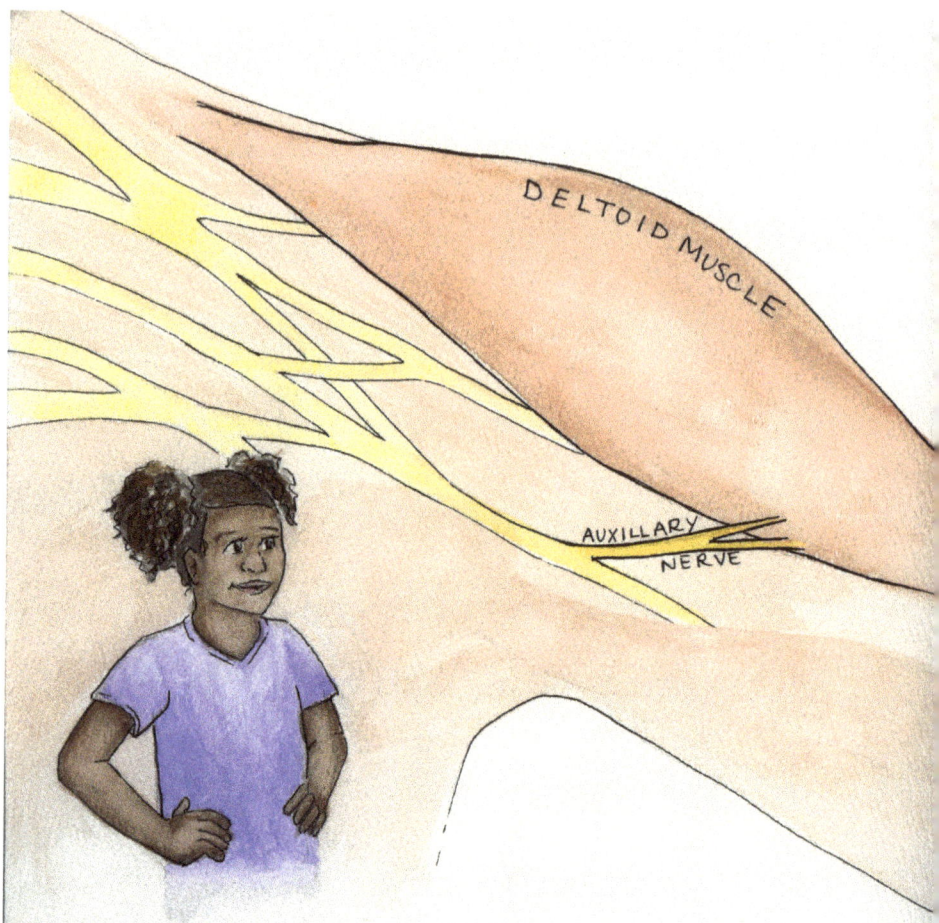

A IS FOR AXILLARY. THE AXILLARY NERVE IS THE BRANCH OF THE BRACHIAL PLEXUS THAT SENDS MESSAGES TO THE DELTOID MUSCLE TO LIFT THE SHOULDER INTO THE AIR.

A IS FOR AXONOTMESIS. AXONOTMESIS IS AN INJURY TO THE NERVE AXON THAT LEAVES THE NERVE PARTIALLY INTACT. AN AXON IS THE NERVE FIBER THAT EXTENDS FROM THE BODY OF THE NERVE CELL AND CARRIES THE MESSAGES FROM THE NERVE TO THE MUSCLE. SURGICAL REPAIR MAY OR MAY NOT BE REQUIRED.

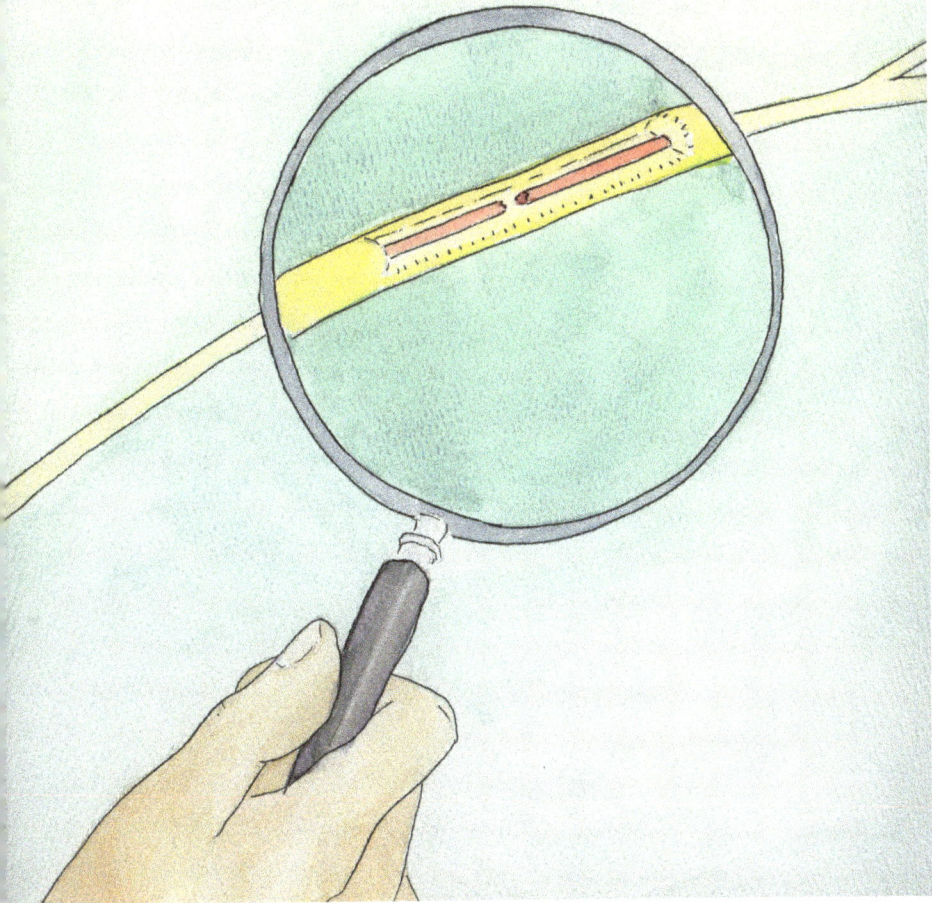

ABCs OF THE BRACHIAL PLEXUS

B IS FOR BELLY TIME. BELLY TIME HELPS GIVE THE WEAK ARM A CHANCE TO STRETCH, GET STRONGER, AND IMPROVES HEAD CONTROL. REMEMBER—BACK-TO-SLEEP AND SUPERVISED BELLY-TO-PLAY.

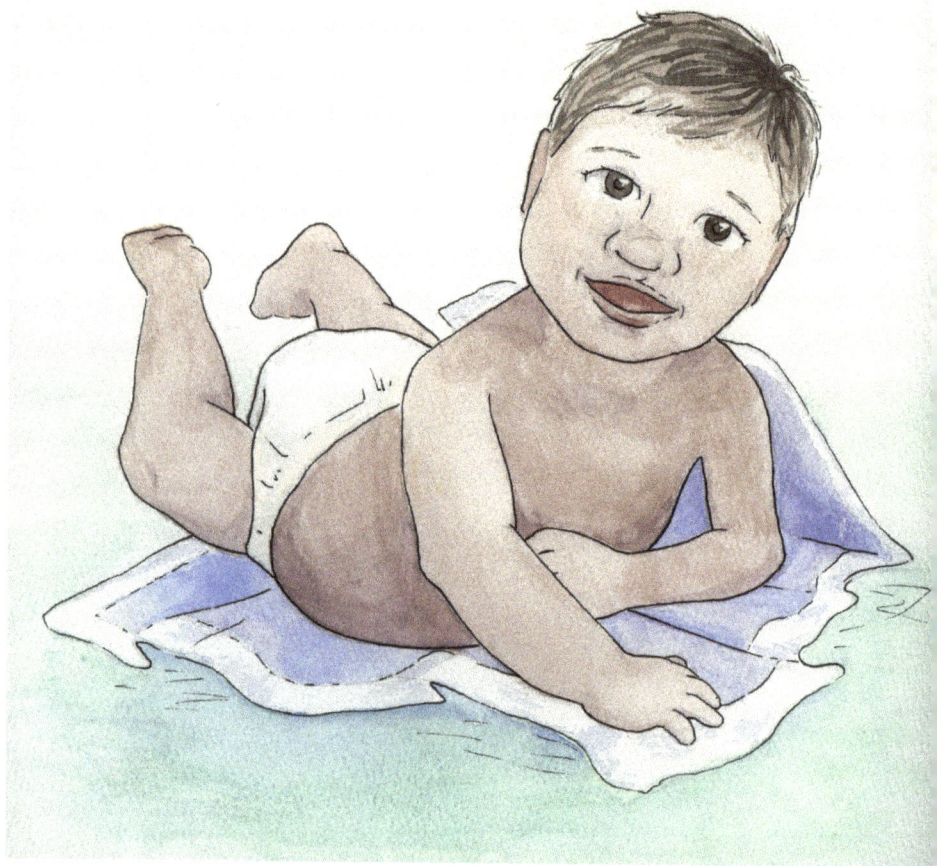

ABCs OF THE BRACHIAL PLEXUS

B IS FOR BENEDICTION SIGN. BENEDICTION SIGN IS A POSTURING OF THE HAND WHEN TRYING TO MAKE A FIST THAT HAPPENS WHEN THERE IS AN INTERRUPTION IN THE SIGNAL TO THE MEDIAN NERVE.

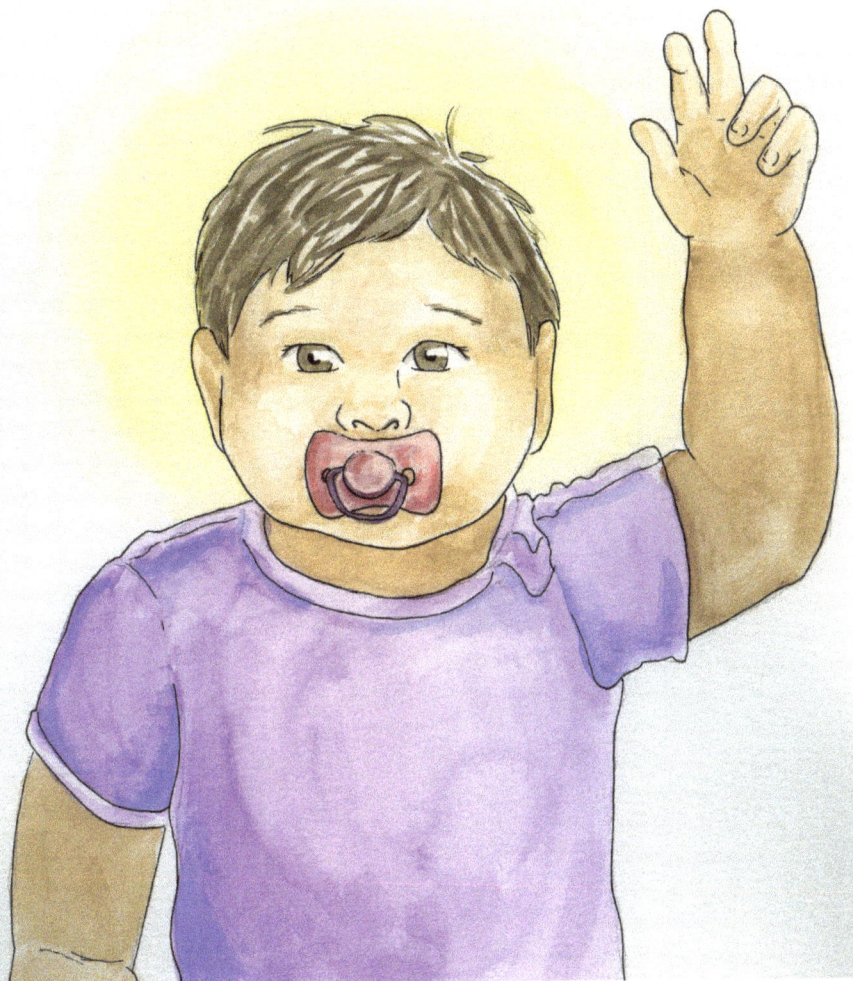

ABCs OF THE BRACHIAL PLEXUS

B IS FOR BICEPS. THE BICEPS IS THE MUSCLE THAT BENDS THE ELBOW. SURGERY MAY NOT BE NEEDED IF A BABY CAN BEND THE ELBOW AT 3 TO 9 MONTHS OF AGE.

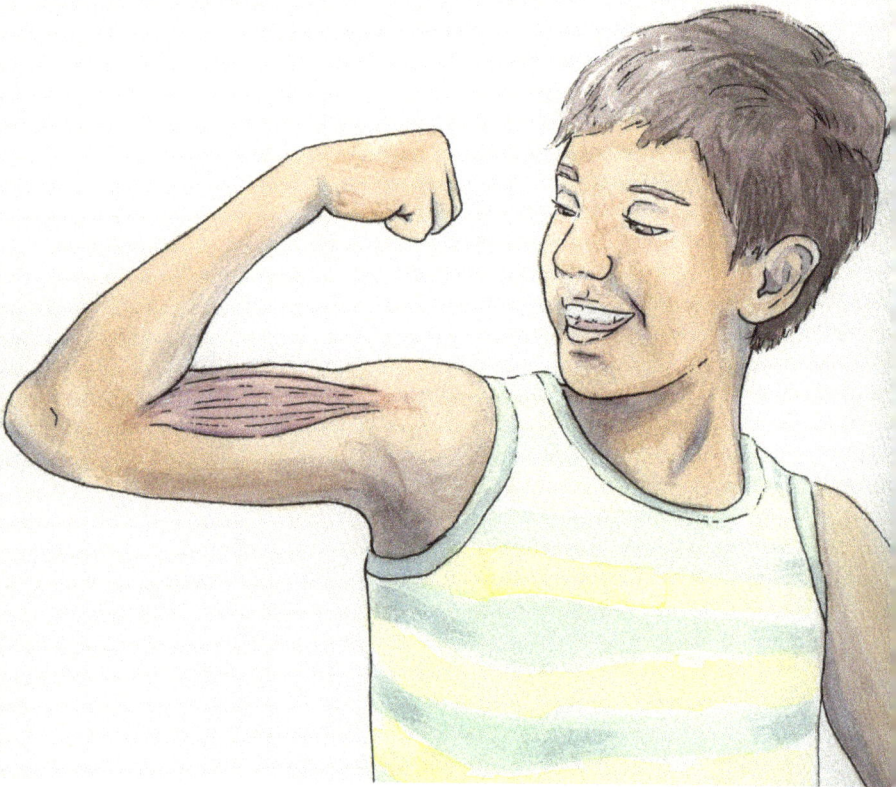

B IS FOR BRACHIAL PLEXUS. THE BRACHIAL PLEXUS IS A COLLECTION OF NERVES THAT SUPPLY MESSAGES TO THE ARM TO MOVE AND FEEL. THE BRACHIAL PLEXUS STARTS WITH THE C5, C6, C7, C8, AND T1 NERVE ROOTS AT THE SPINAL CORD, AND ENDS WITH THE AXILLARY, RADIAL, MUSCULOCUTANEOUS, ULNAR, AND MEDIAN NERVE BRANCHES.

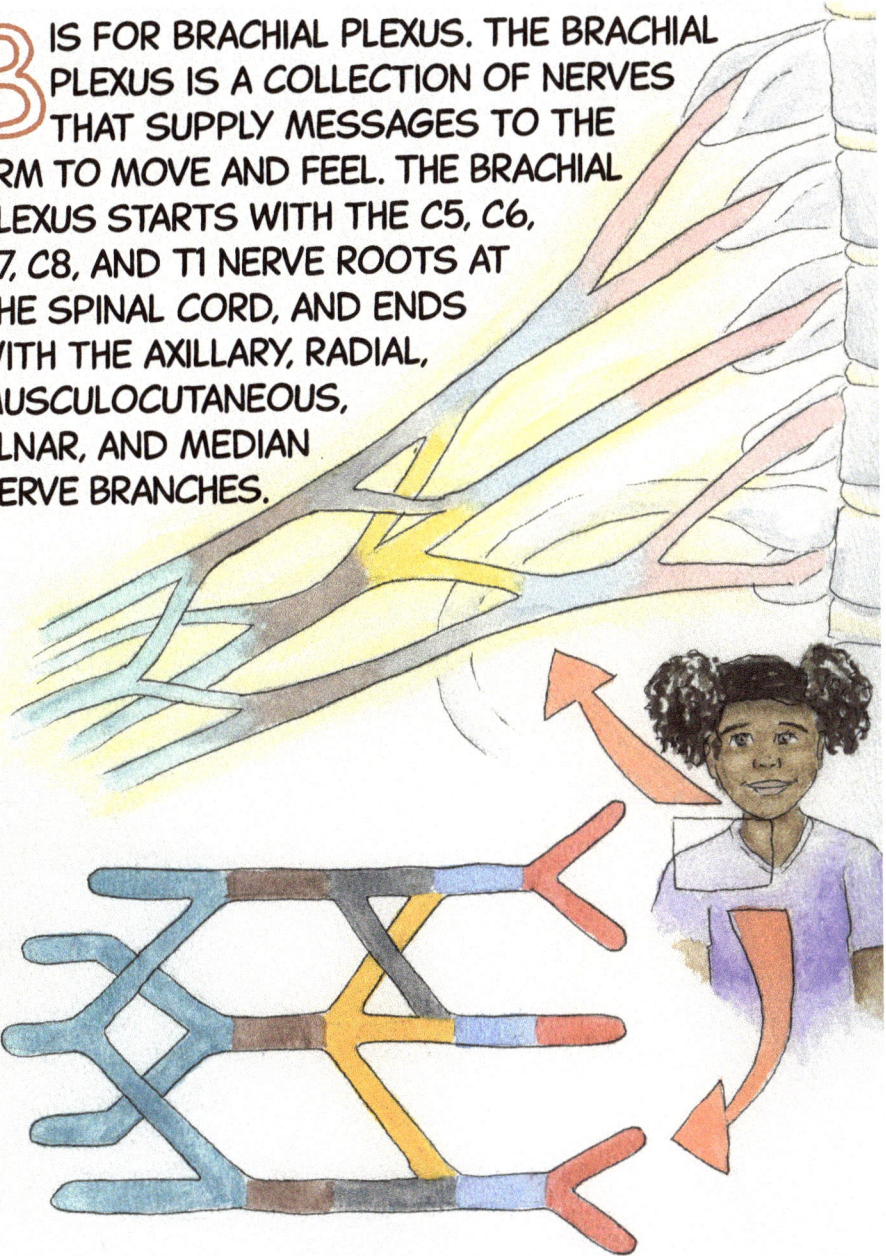

B IS FOR BRACING. BRACING IS USED TO PROTECT THE ARM AND INCISION AFTER SURGERY, AND MAY BE NEEDED FOR UP TO 6 WEEKS.

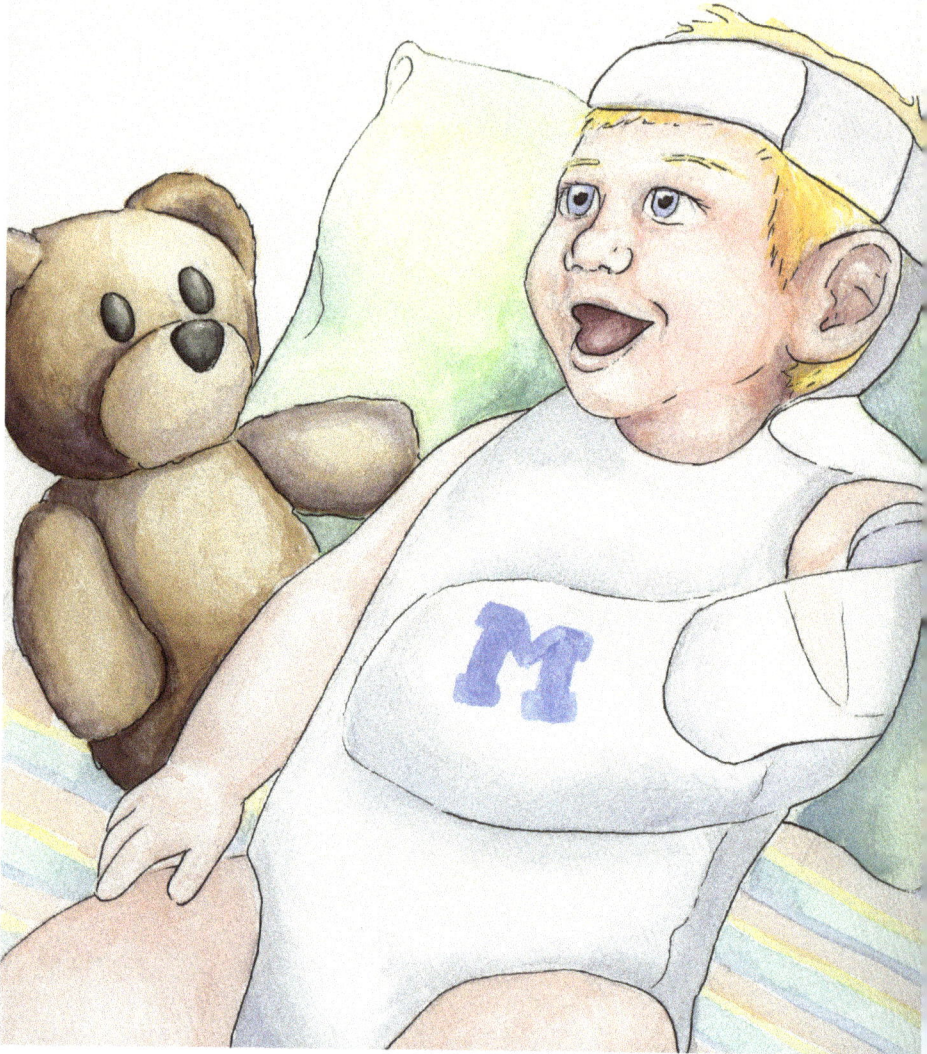

ABCs OF THE BRACHIAL PLEXUS

B IS FOR BRANCHES. BRANCHES OF THE BRACHIAL PLEXUS ARE THE NERVES FARTHEST FROM THE SPINE THAT CONNECT TO THE MUSCLES. THE TERMINAL BRANCHES INCLUDE MUSCULOCUTANEOUS, AXILLARY, MEDIAN, RADIAL, AND ULNAR NERVES.

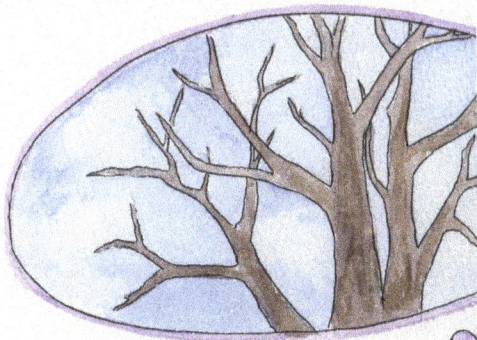

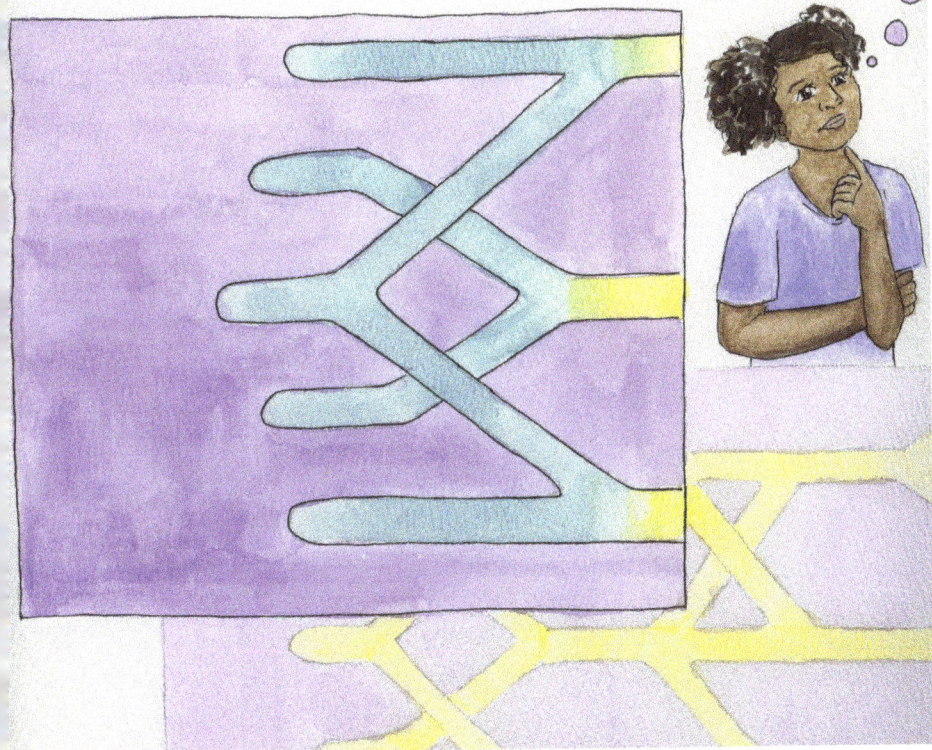

ABCs OF THE BRACHIAL PLEXUS

C IS FOR CAST. CASTS ARE USED TO IMMOBILIZE A JOINT AFTER SHOULDER OR ELBOW SURGERY.

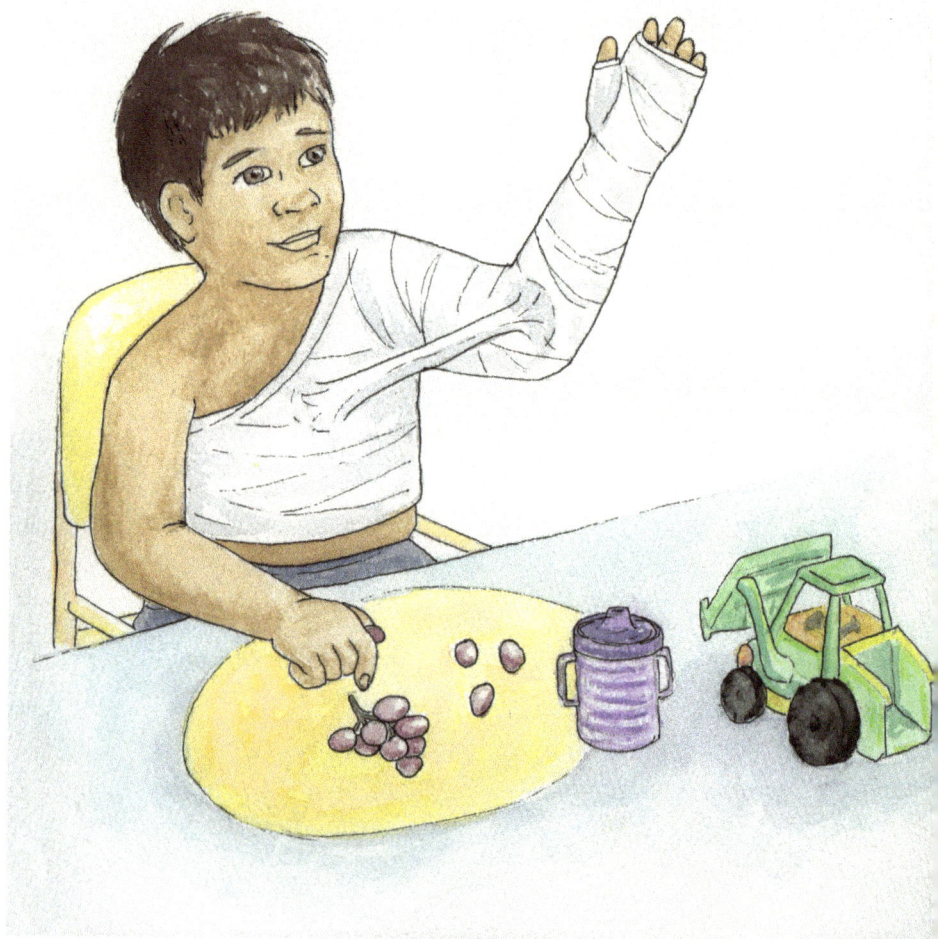

ABCs OF THE BRACHIAL PLEXUS

C IS FOR CERVICAL. CERVICAL COMES FROM THE LATIN TERM FOR NECK. CERVICAL NERVES 5, 6, 7, AND 8 ARE PART OF THE BRACHIAL PLEXUS.

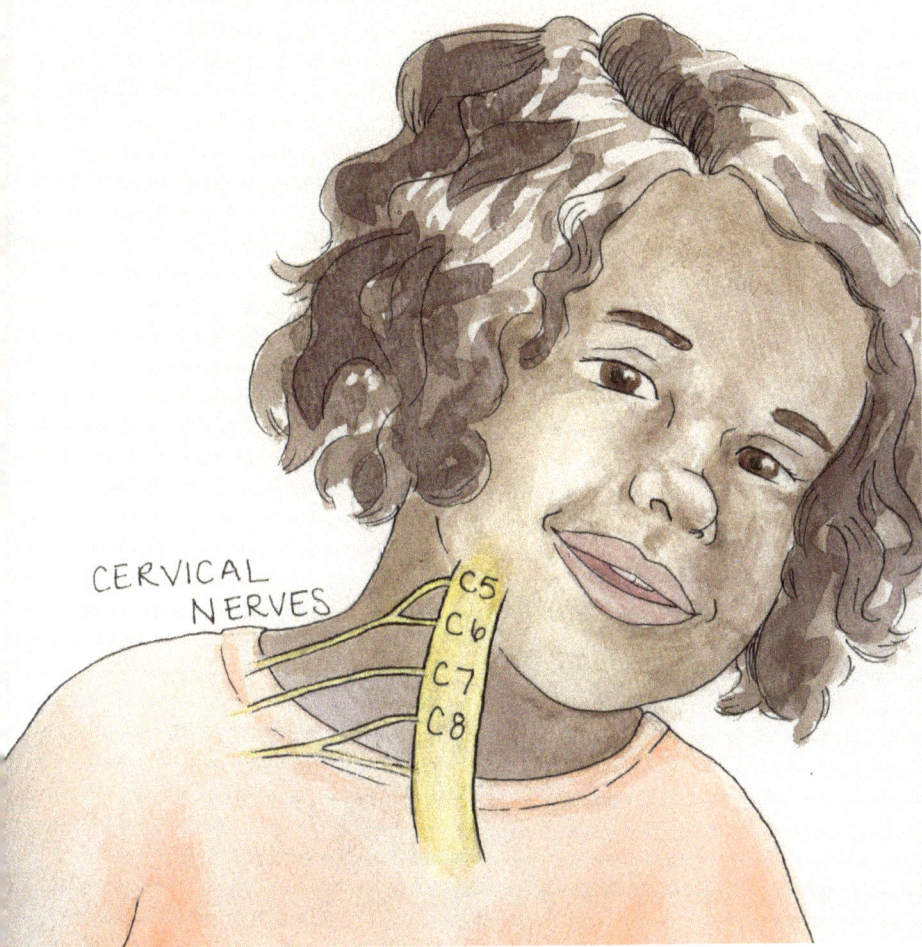

CERVICAL NERVES

C5
C6
C7
C8

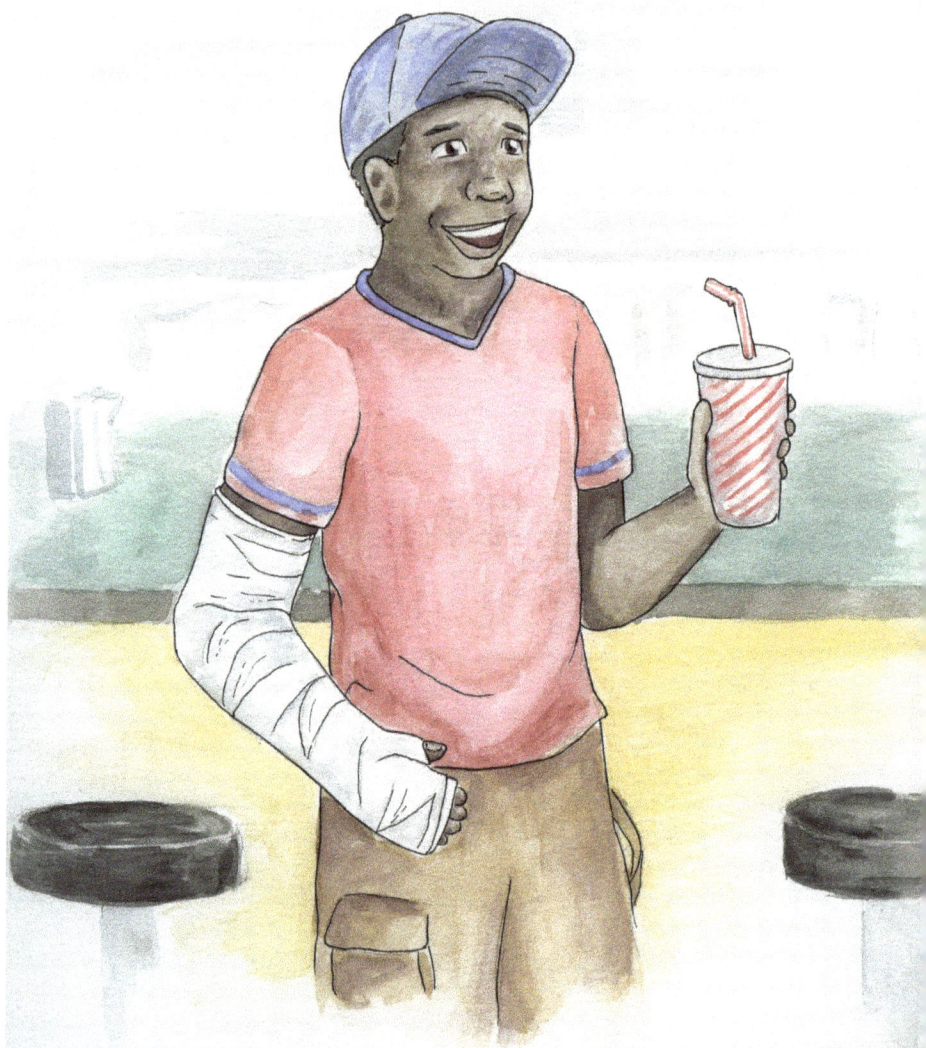

C IS FOR CONSTRAINT THERAPY.
CONSTRAINT THERAPY INCLUDES THE USE OF A CAST ON THE STRONGER ARM TO HELP THE WEAKER ARM IMPROVE.

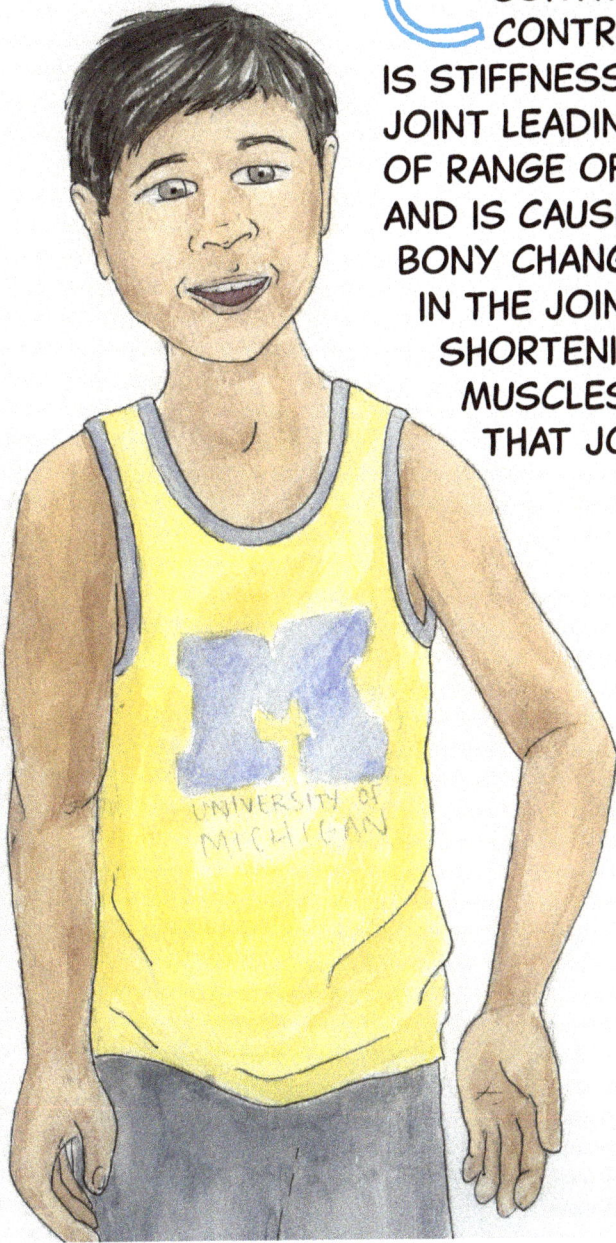

C IS FOR CONTRACTURE. CONTRACTURE IS STIFFNESS IN THE JOINT LEADING TO LACK OF RANGE OF MOTION, AND IS CAUSED BY BONY CHANGES IN THE JOINT OR SHORTENING OF THE MUSCLES AROUND THAT JOINT.

C IS FOR CORDS. THE BRACHIAL PLEXUS CONTAINS THE LATERAL, POSTERIOR, AND MEDIAL CORDS THAT ARE CREATED WHEN THE 6 NERVE DIVISIONS COME TOGETHER.

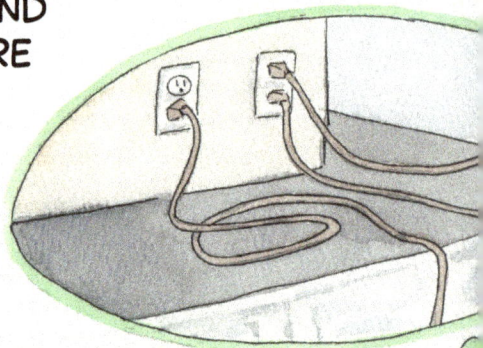

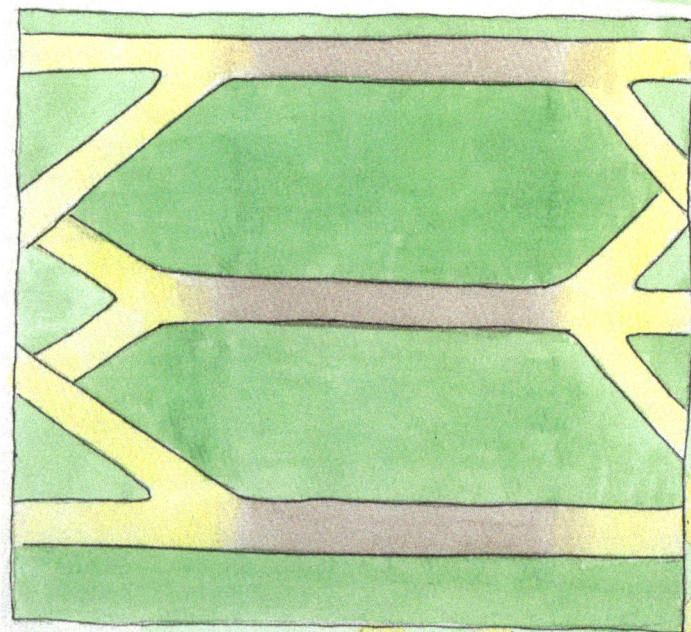

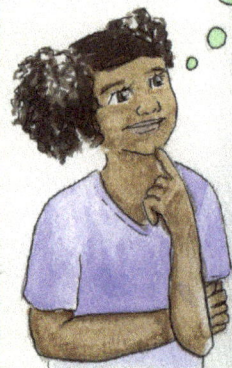

D IS FOR DEXTERITY. DEXTERITY IS THE ABILITY TO USE THE SMALL MUSCLES OF THE HAND TO MANIPULATE OBJECTS.

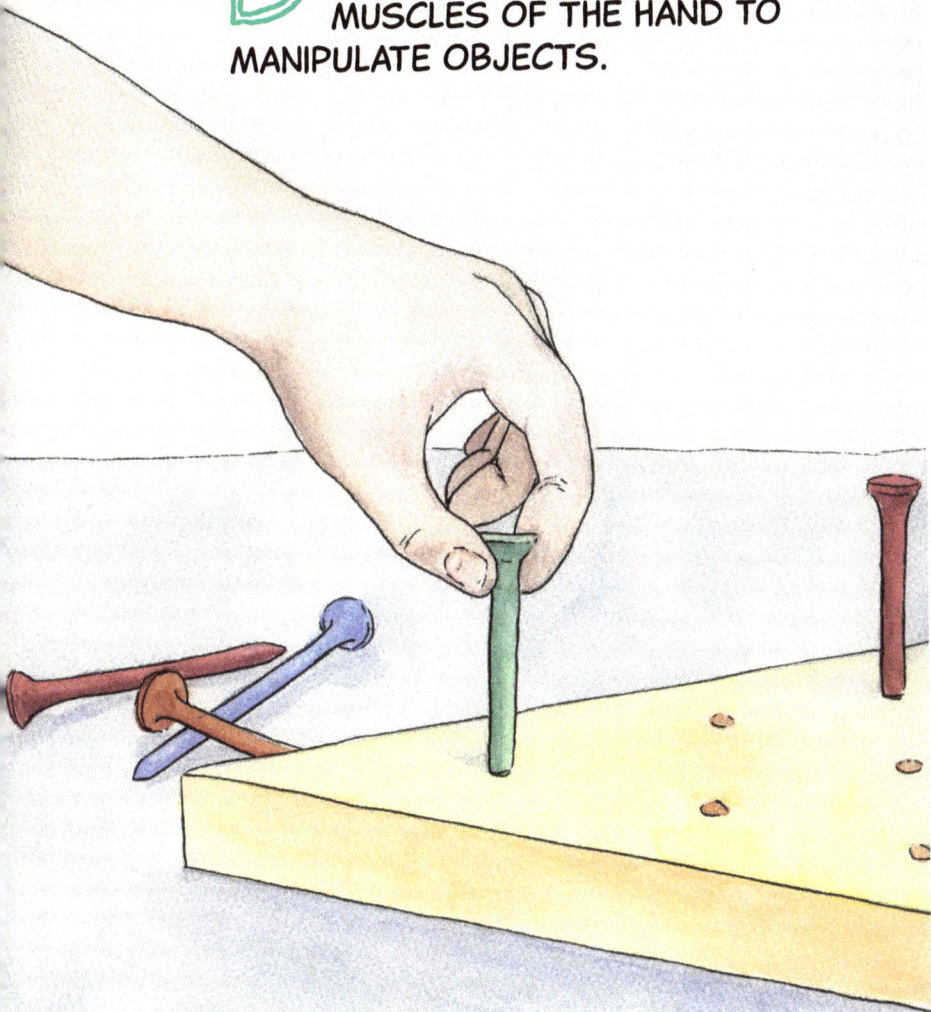

D IS FOR DIAGNOSTIC TESTS. DIAGNOSTIC TESTS MAY BE RECOMMENDED TO HELP EVALUATE THE EXTENT AND SEVERITY OF STRETCH TO THE BRACHIAL PLEXUS. SOME OF THE DIAGNOSTIC TESTS INCLUDE ELECTRODIAGNOSTIC (EDX) TESTS THAT ARE USED TO ASSESS THE CONTINUITY AND FUNCTION OF A NERVE, MAGNETIC RESONANCE IMAGING (MRI), AND COMPUTED TOMOGRAPHY MYELOGRAM (CTM).

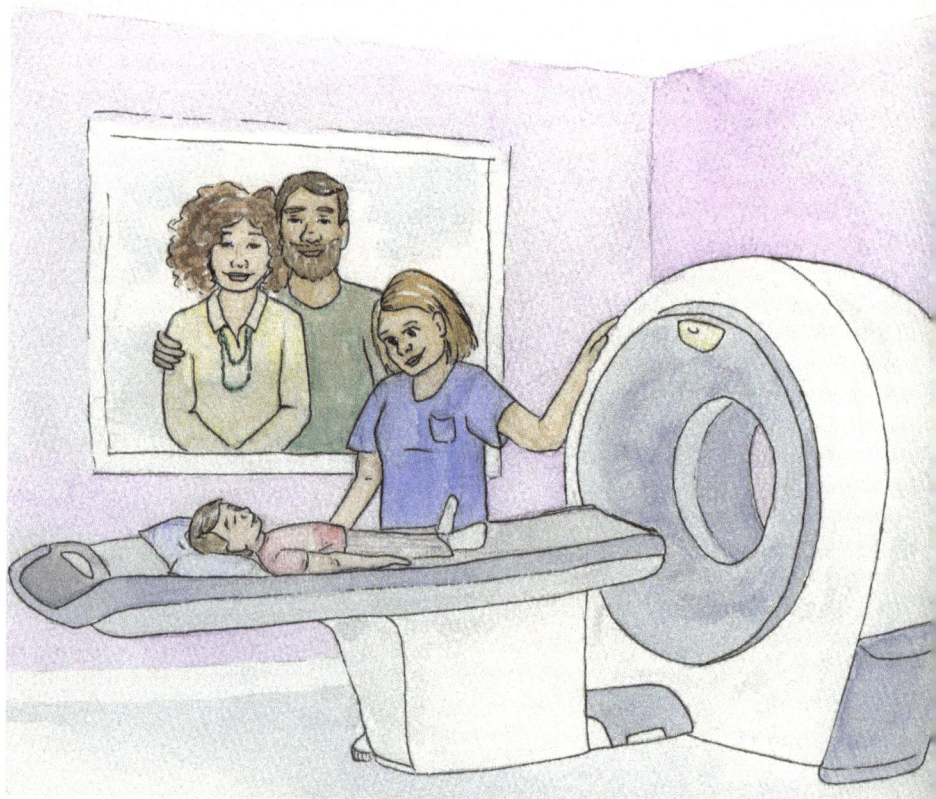

D IS FOR DIVISIONS. THERE ARE 6 DIVISIONS OF THE BRACHIAL PLEXUS, WHICH INCLUDE THE ANTERIOR AND POSTERIOR PORTIONS OF THE SUPERIOR (UPPER), MIDDLE, AND INFERIOR (LOWER) TRUNKS.

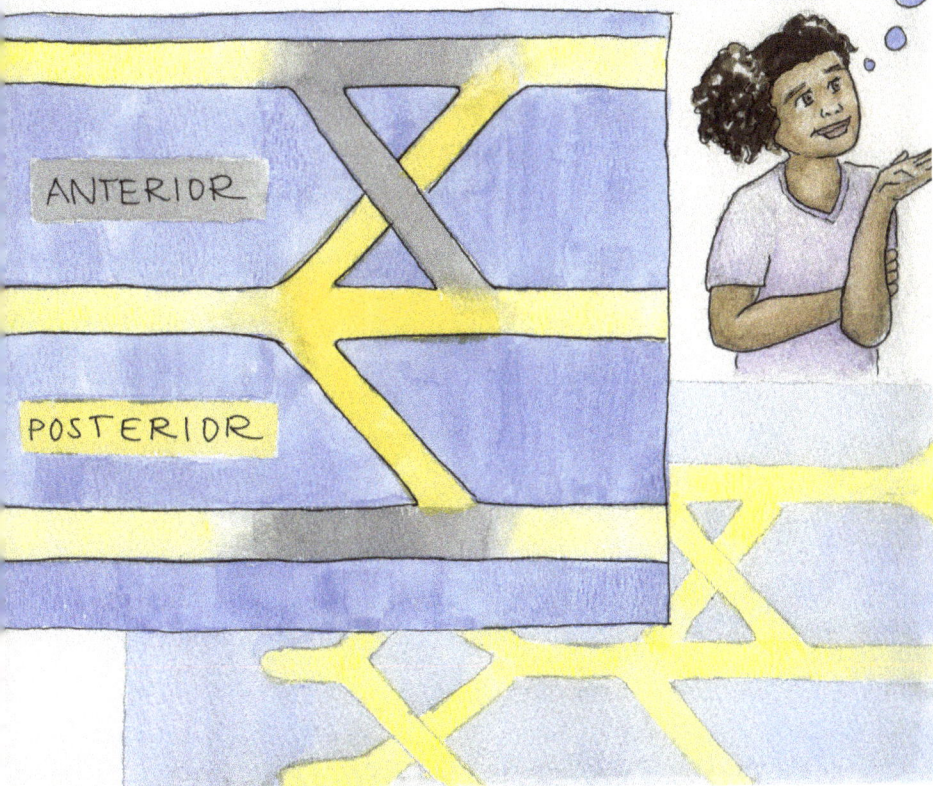

ABCs OF THE BRACHIAL PLEXUS

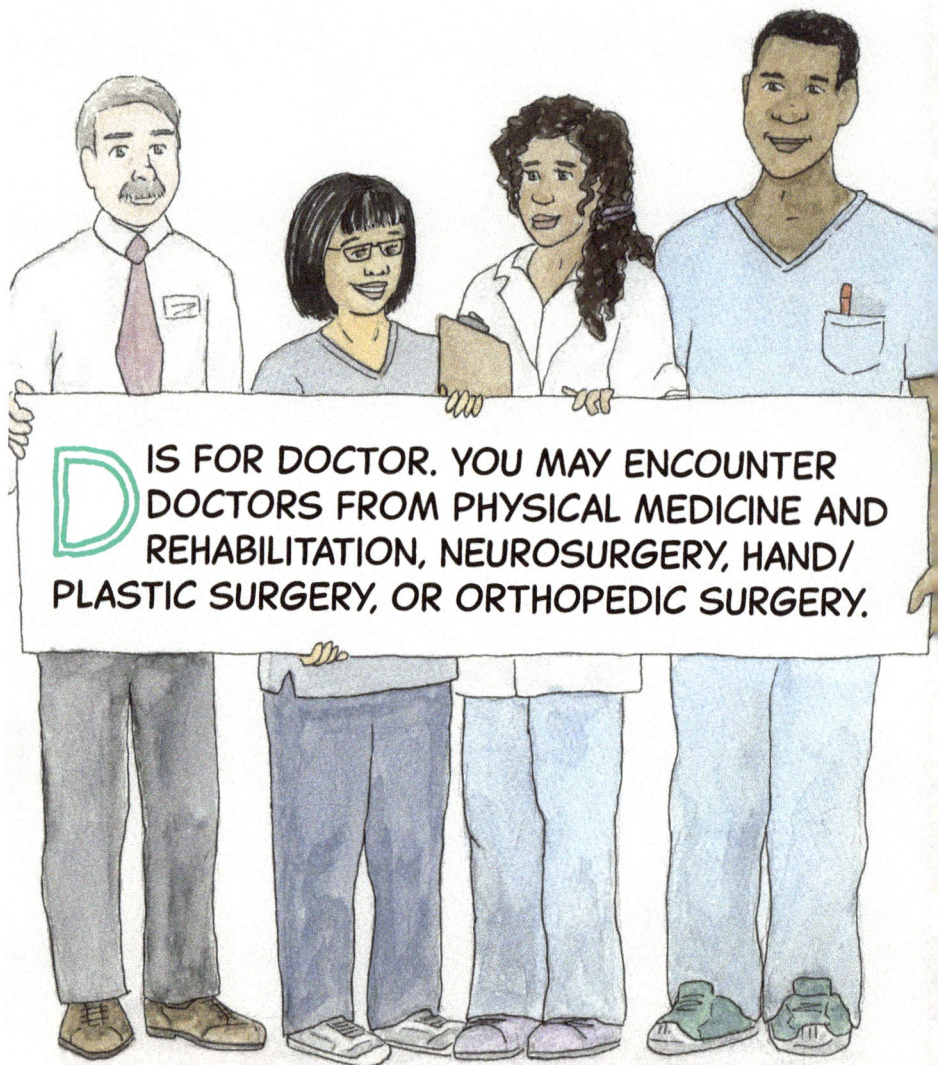

D IS FOR DOCTOR. YOU MAY ENCOUNTER DOCTORS FROM PHYSICAL MEDICINE AND REHABILITATION, NEUROSURGERY, HAND/PLASTIC SURGERY, OR ORTHOPEDIC SURGERY.

ABCs OF THE BRACHIAL PLEXUS

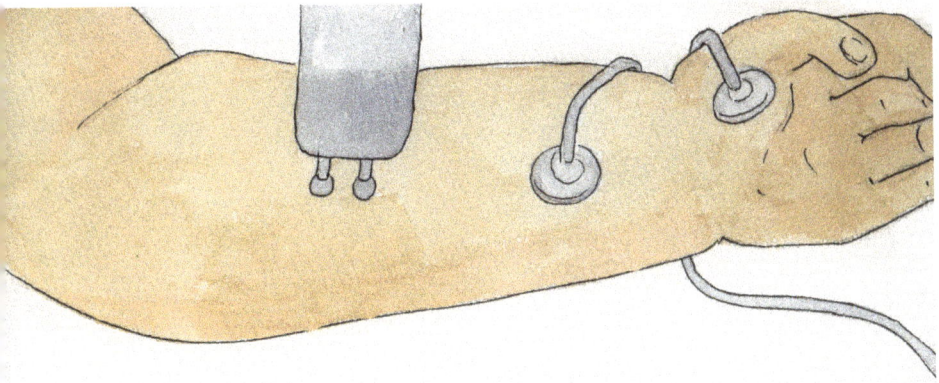

E IS FOR EMG. EMG IS AN ELECTROMYOGRAM. THIS ELECTRODIAGNOSTIC TEST IS PERFORMED AT LEAST 1 MONTH AFTER ONSET OF NEONATAL BRACHIAL PLEXUS PALSY. TESTING INVOLVES THE USE OF SMALL ELECTRODES THAT CAN DETECT MUSCLE ACTIVITY.

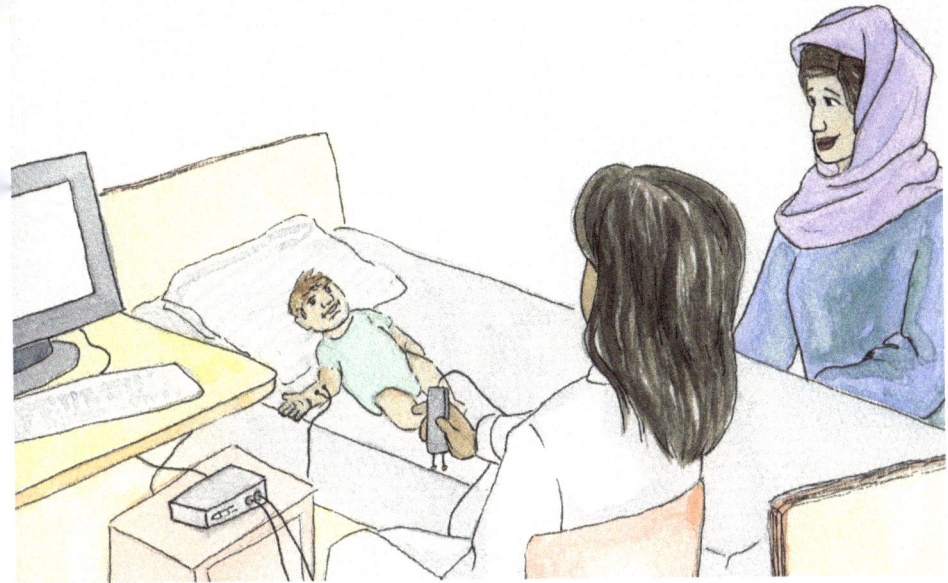

ABCs OF THE BRACHIAL PLEXUS

E IS FOR ERB'S PALSY. ERB'S PALSY IS A TERM USED TO DESCRIBE THE TYPE OF NEONATAL BRACHIAL PLEXUS PALSY THAT INVOLVES THE UPPER 2 OR 3 NERVES—C5, C6, AND SOMETIMES C7. THIS IS THE MOST COMMON TYPE OF NEONATAL BRACHIAL PLEXUS PALSY.

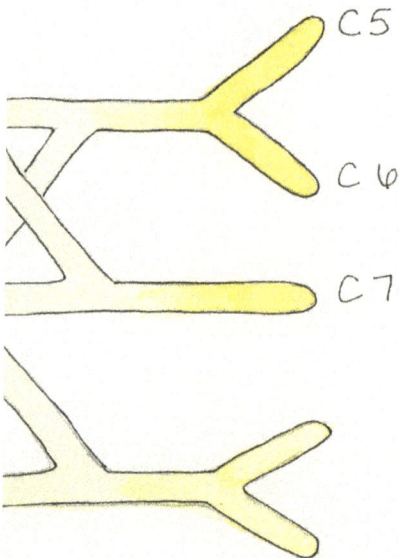

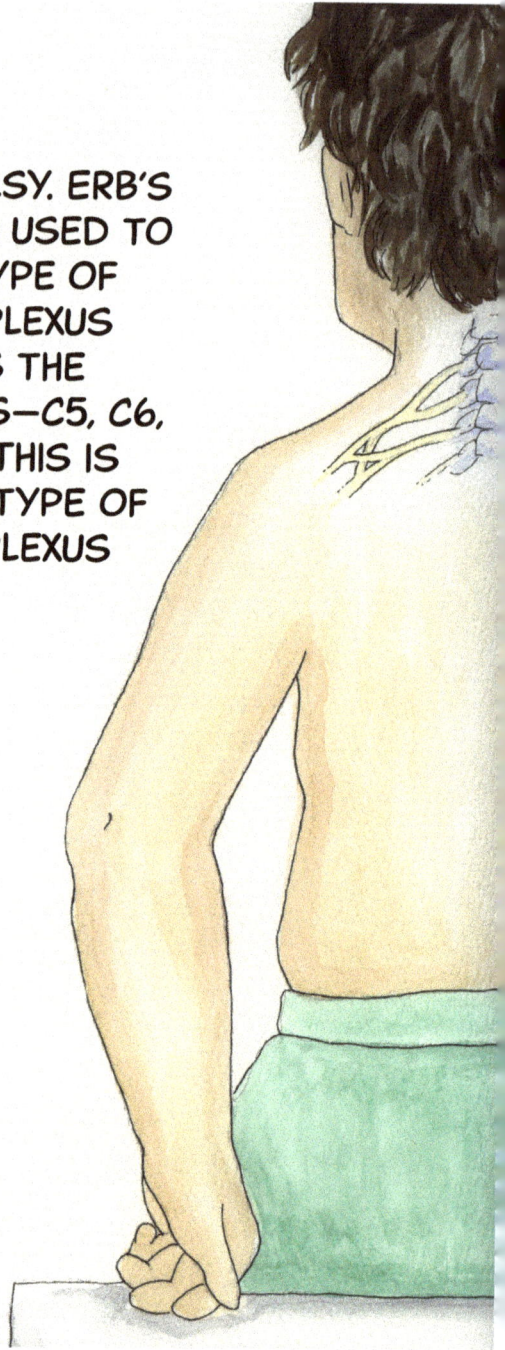

C5

C6

C7

ABCs OF THE BRACHIAL PLEXUS

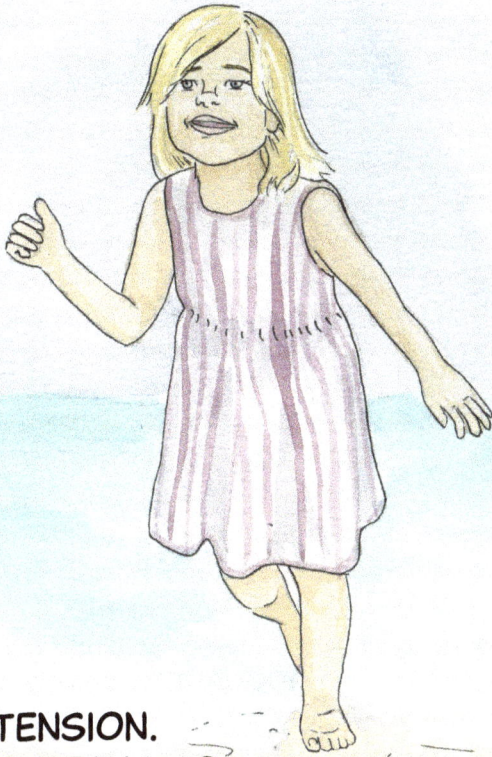

E IS FOR EXTENSION.
EXTENSION MEANS TO
STRAIGHTEN THE JOINT.

F IS FOR FLACCID. FLACCID INDICATES WEAKNESS WITH COMPLETE LACK OF MUSCLE FIRMNESS.

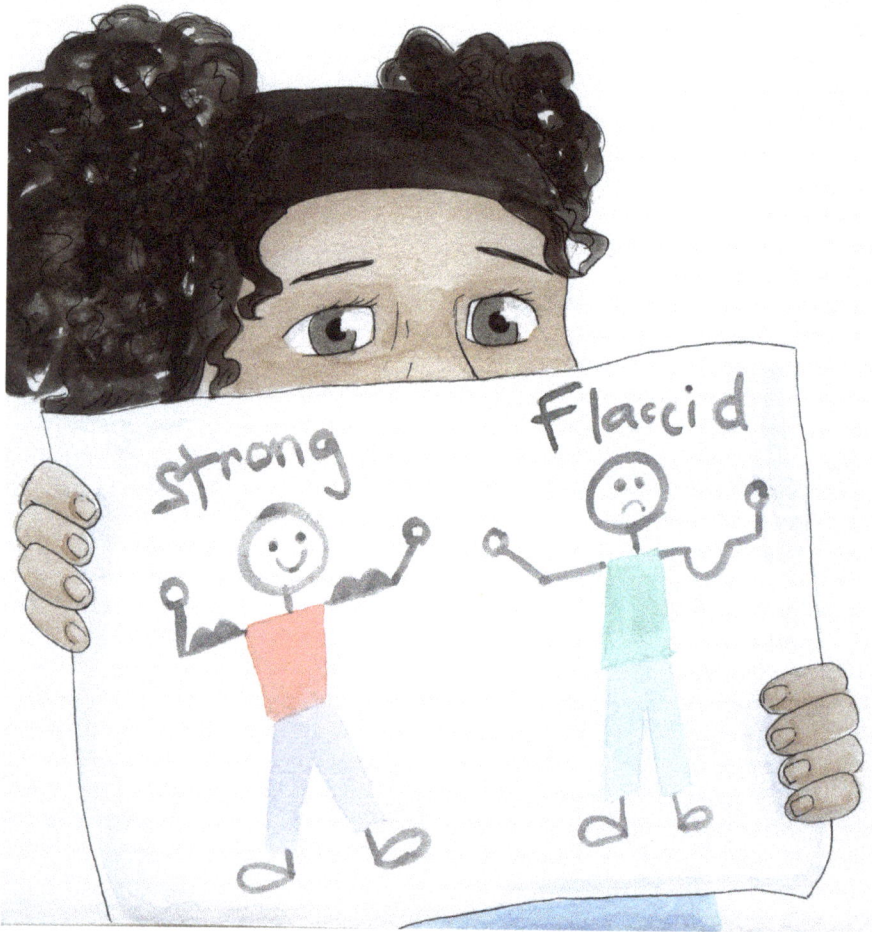

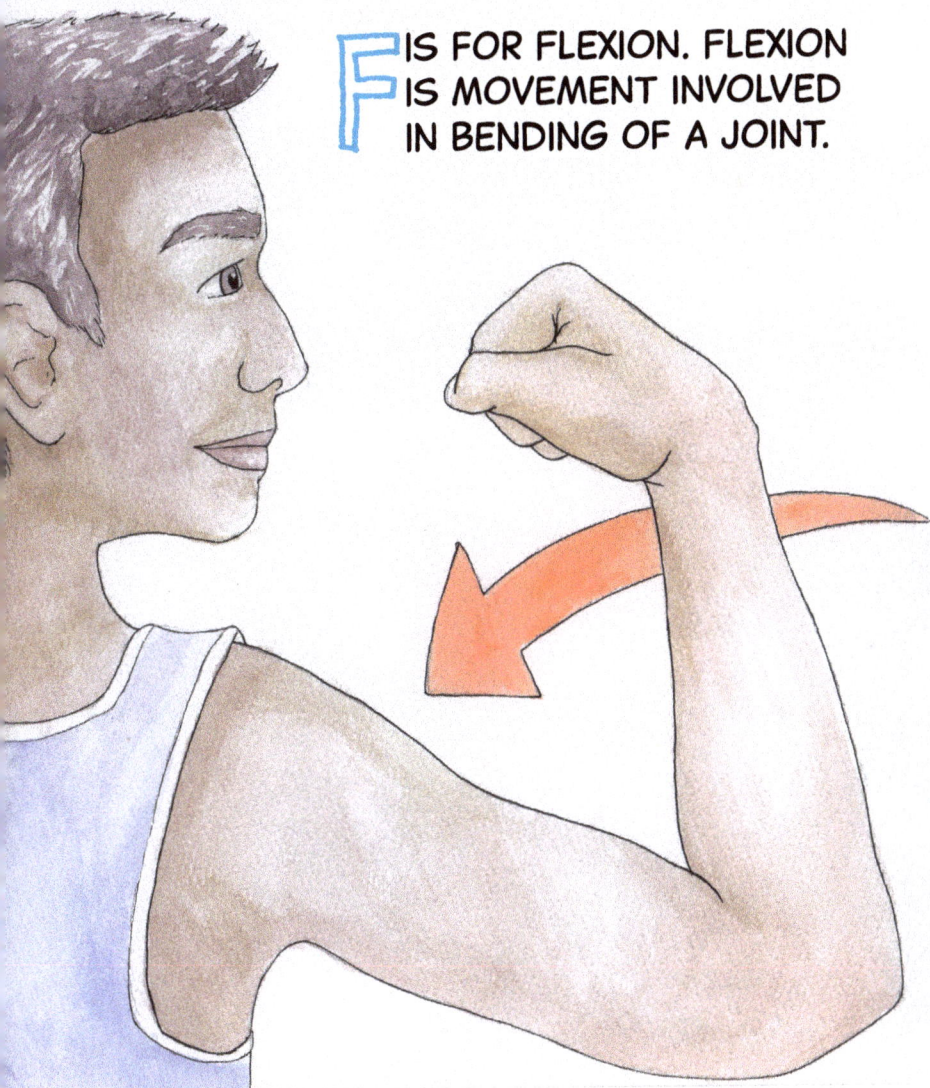

F IS FOR FLEXION. FLEXION IS MOVEMENT INVOLVED IN BENDING OF A JOINT.

G IS FOR GONIOMETER. A GONIOMETER IS A TOOL THAT MEASURES THE AMOUNT OF MOTION THERE IS IN EACH JOINT.

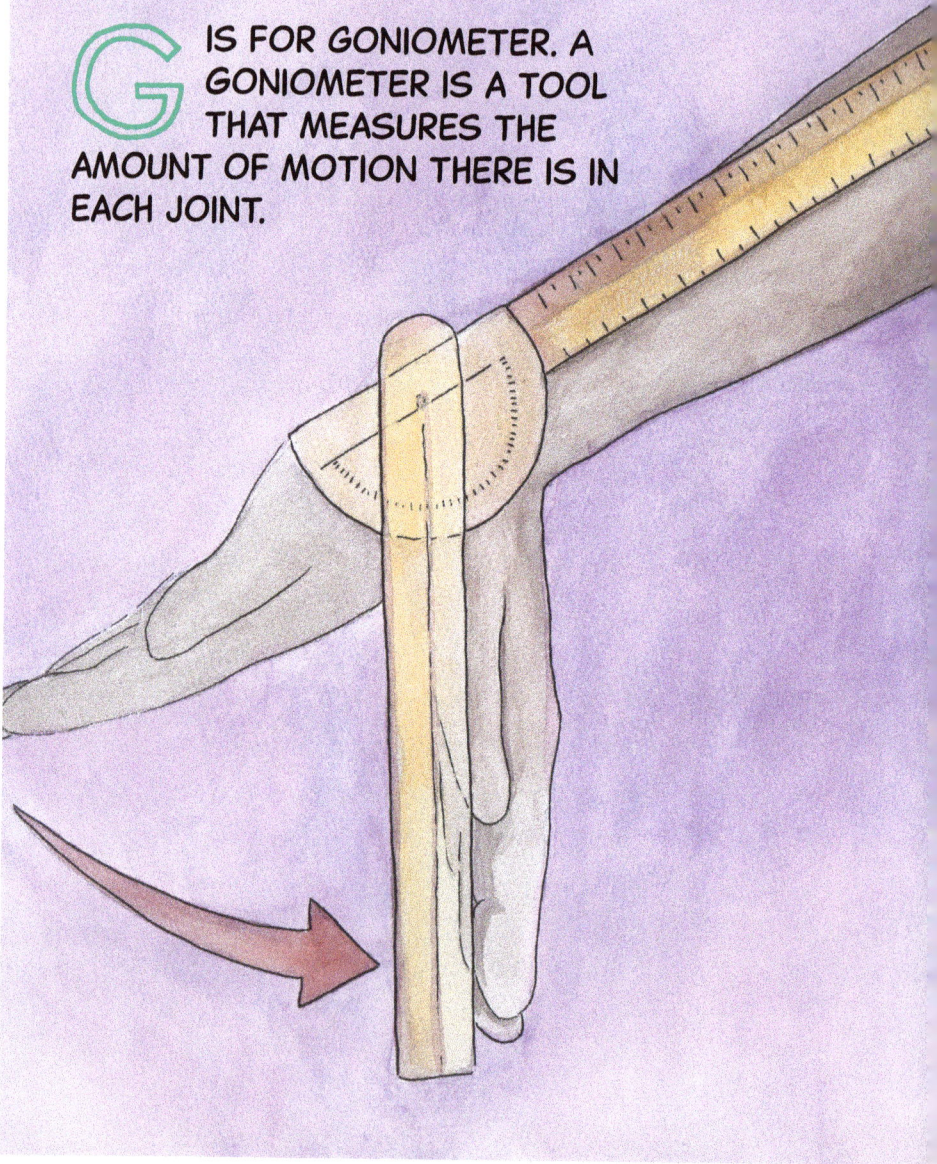

ABCs OF THE BRACHIAL PLEXUS

G IS FOR GRIEVING. GRIEVING IS COMMON FOR PARENTS WHEN THEY REALIZE THEIR CHILD'S ARM IS NOT WORKING FULLY, AND IT IS UNKNOWN HOW MUCH MOTION THE CHILD WILL REGAIN.

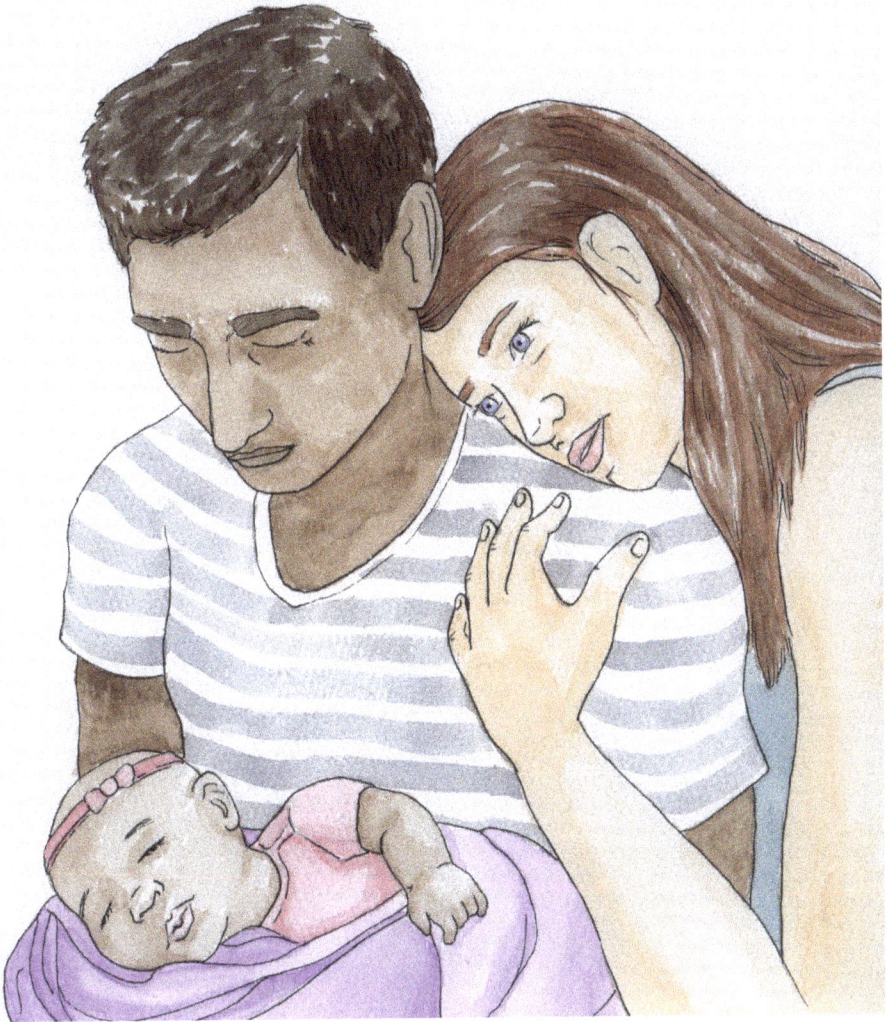

H IS FOR HORNER'S SYNDROME. HORNER'S SYNDROME IS A DROOPY EYE, A LACK OF SWEATING ON THE FACE, AND THE INABILITY OF THE PUPIL TO ENLARGE. THESE SYMPTOMS ALL OCCUR ON THE SAME SIDE AS THE NEONATAL BRACHIAL PLEXUS PALSY.

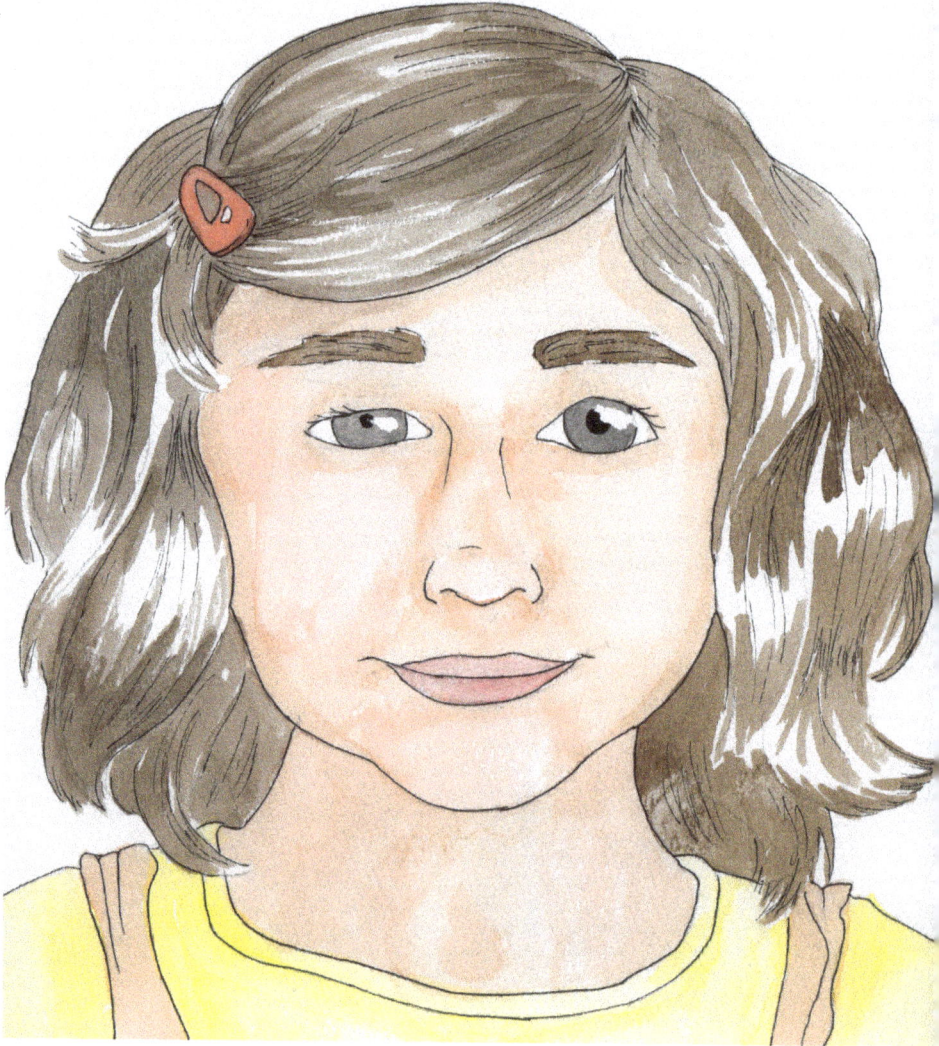

ABCs OF THE BRACHIAL PLEXUS

1 to 4 cases of

BPP for

every...

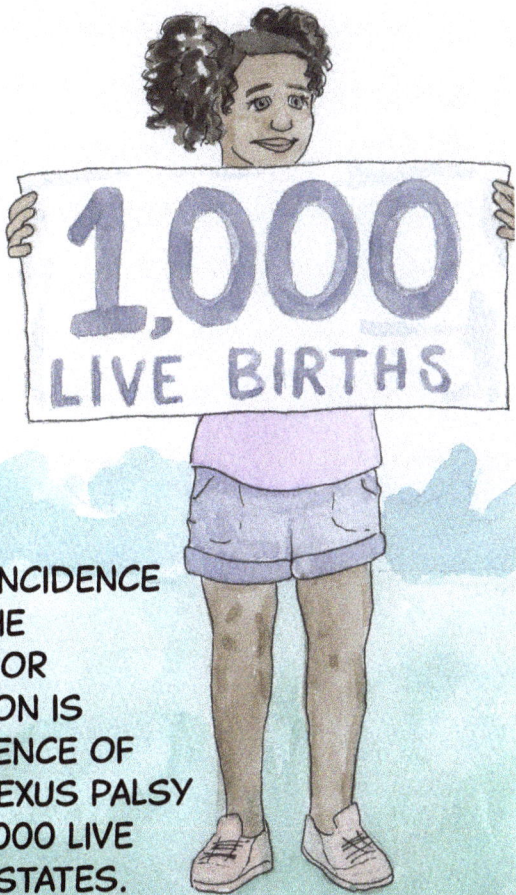

1,000
LIVE BIRTHS

I IS FOR INCIDENCE. INCIDENCE IS A MEASURE OF THE OCCURRENCE, RATE, OR FREQUENCY A CONDITION IS DIAGNOSED. THE INCIDENCE OF NEONATAL BRACHIAL PLEXUS PALSY IS 1 TO 4 CASES PER 1,000 LIVE BIRTHS IN THE UNITED STATES.

IS FOR INNERVATION.
INNERVATION MEANS
THAT MESSAGES
ARE TRAVELING FROM
THE BRAIN TO THE
MUSCLE THROUGH
THE NERVE WITHOUT
INTERRUPTION.

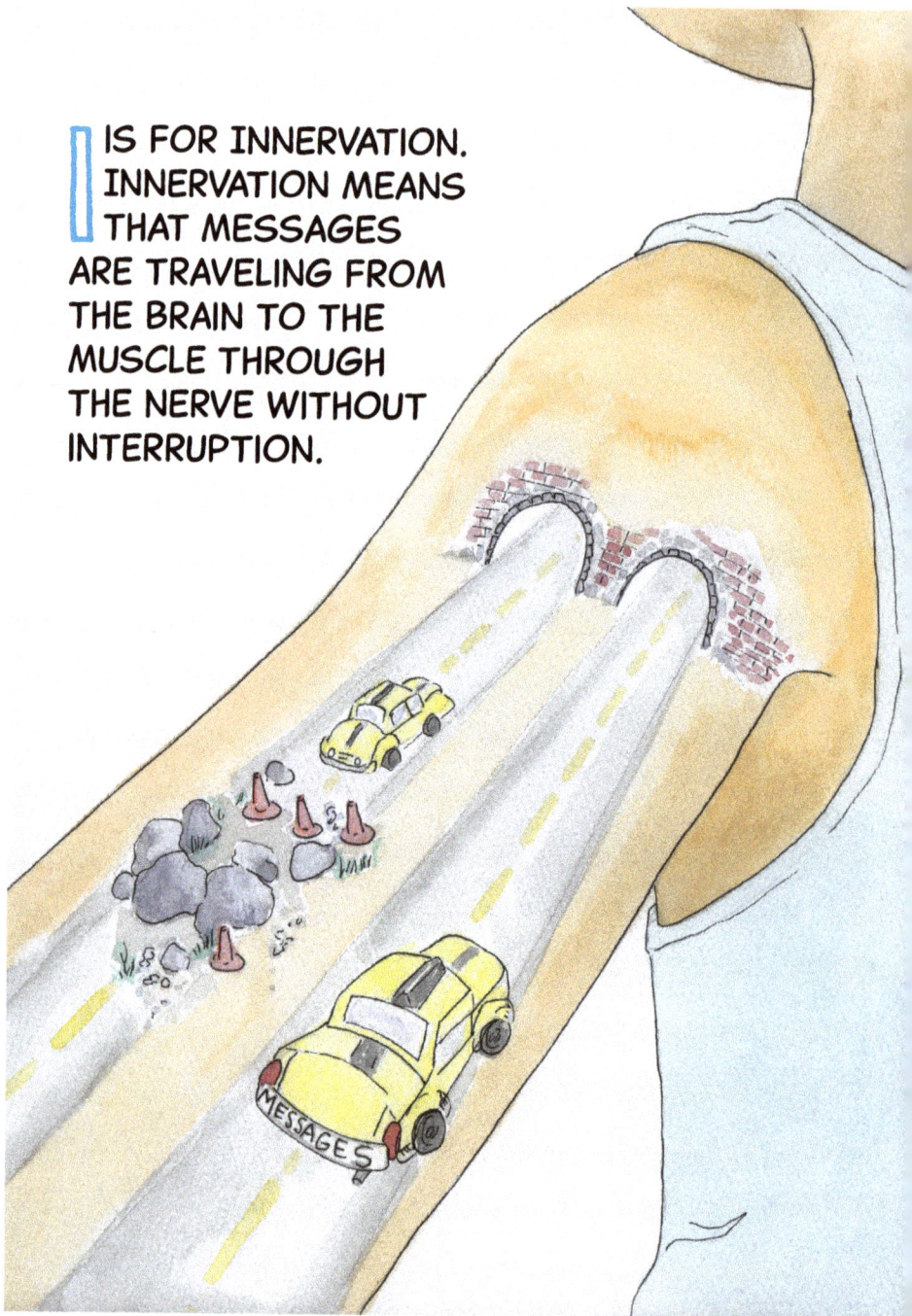

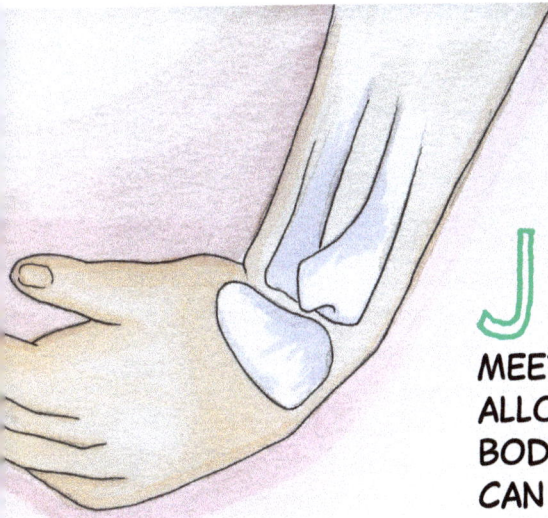

J IS FOR JOINT. A JOINT IS WHERE TWO BODY PARTS MEET TOGETHER TO ALLOW BENDING OF THE BODY PART. A JOINT CAN BECOME TIGHT OR CONTRACTED IF YOU DO NOT STRETCH OR DO EXERCISES.

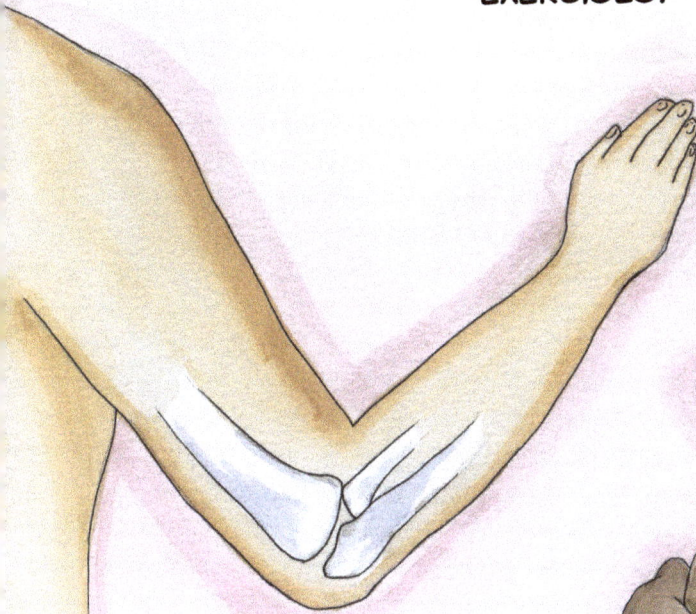

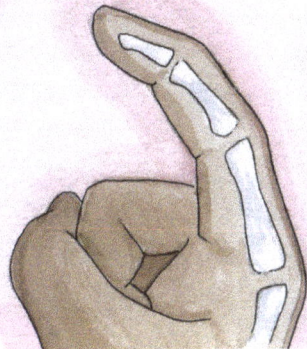

K IS FOR KLUMPKE'S PALSY. KLUMPKE'S PALSY IS THE RAREST FORM OF A NEONATAL BRACHIAL PLEXUS PALSY IN WHICH THE LOWER 2 OR 3 NERVES OF THE BRACHIAL PLEXUS HAVE BEEN STRETCHED, RUPTURED, OR SEPARATED FROM THE SPINAL CORD, CAUSING THE HAND TO BE WEAK.

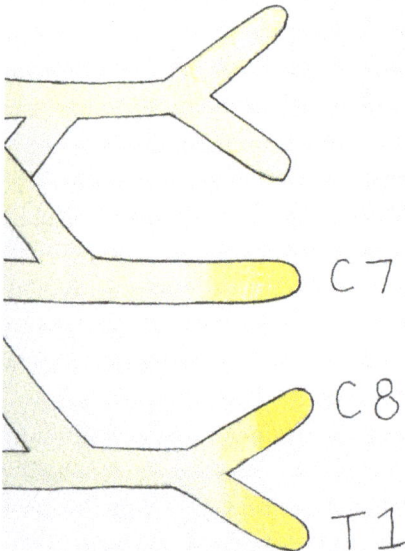

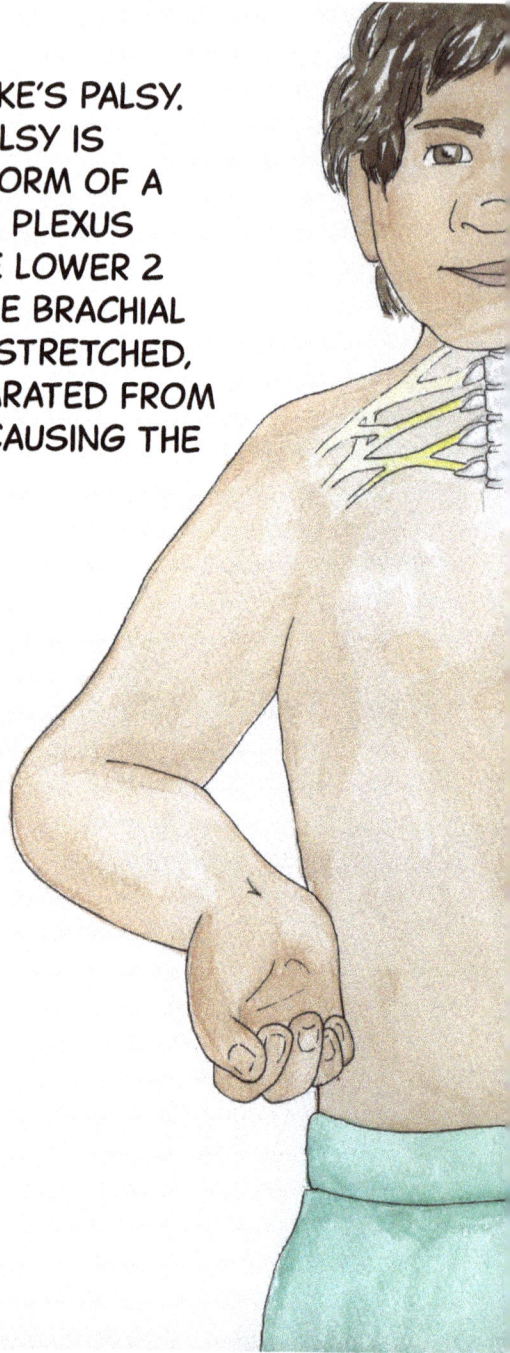

C7

C8

T1

ABCs OF THE BRACHIAL PLEXUS

L

IS FOR LONG-TERM. LONG-TERM AS WELL AS TEMPORARY WEAKNESS CAN OCCUR WITH NEONATAL BRACHIAL PLEXUS PALSY.

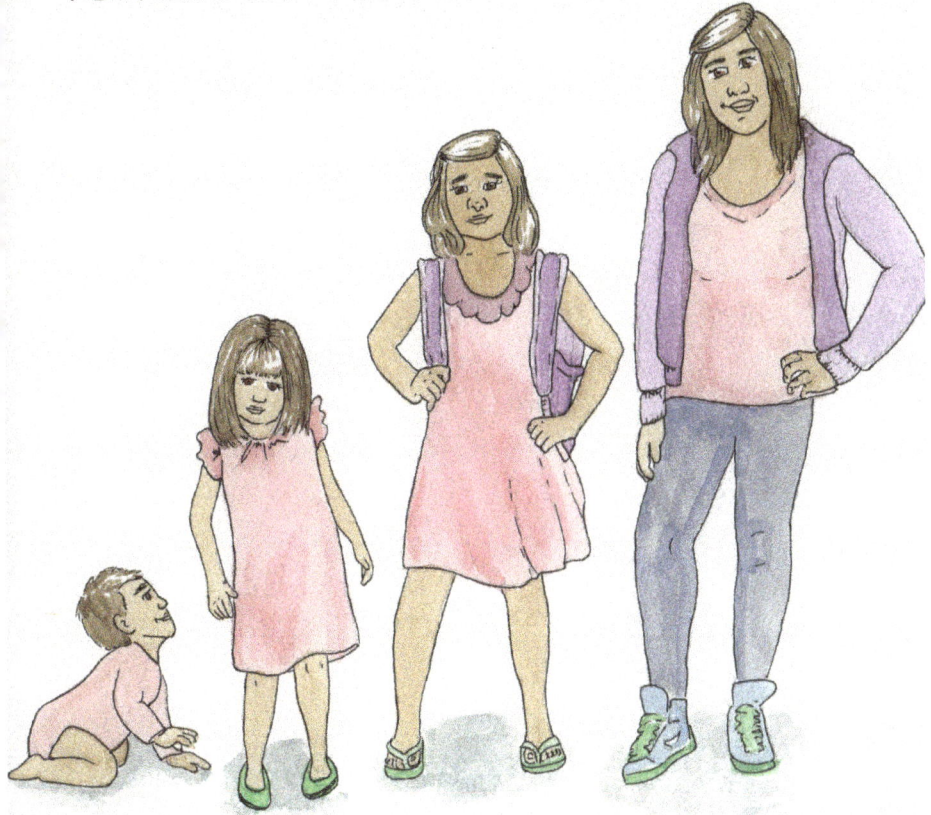

M IS FOR MEDIAN NERVE. THE MEDIAN NERVE IS THE BRANCH OF THE BRACHIAL PLEXUS THAT HELPS CONTROL INWARD FOREARM ROTATION AND THE MUSCLES THAT BEND THE FINGERS, ESPECIALLY THE THUMB, POINTER, AND MIDDLE FINGERS.

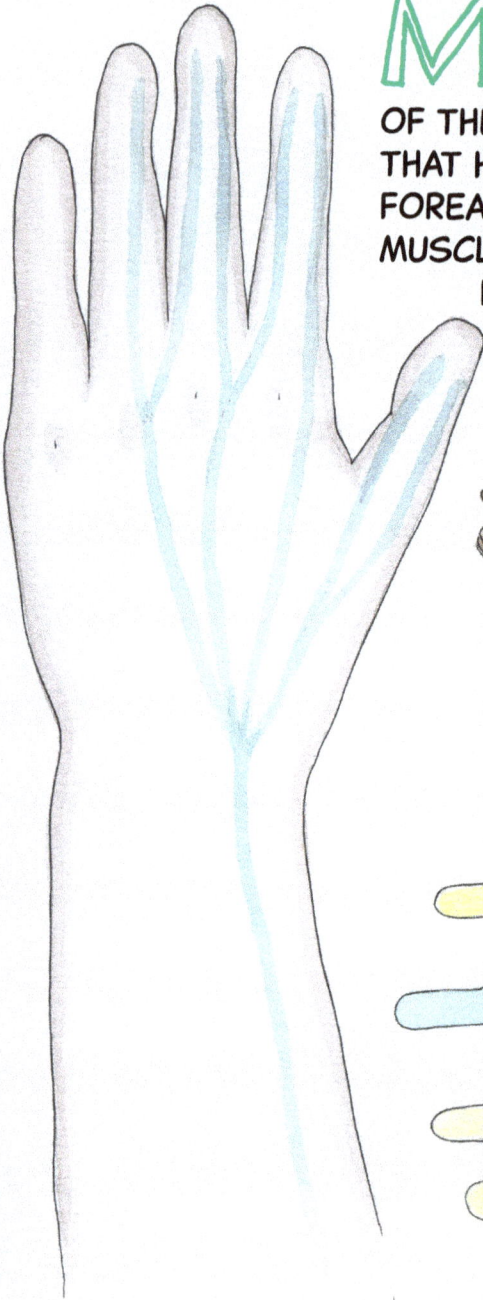

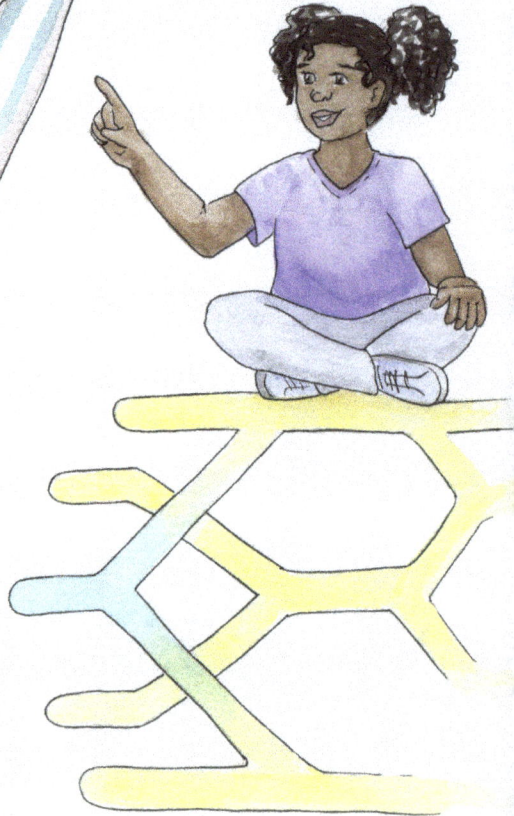

ABCs OF THE BRACHIAL PLEXUS

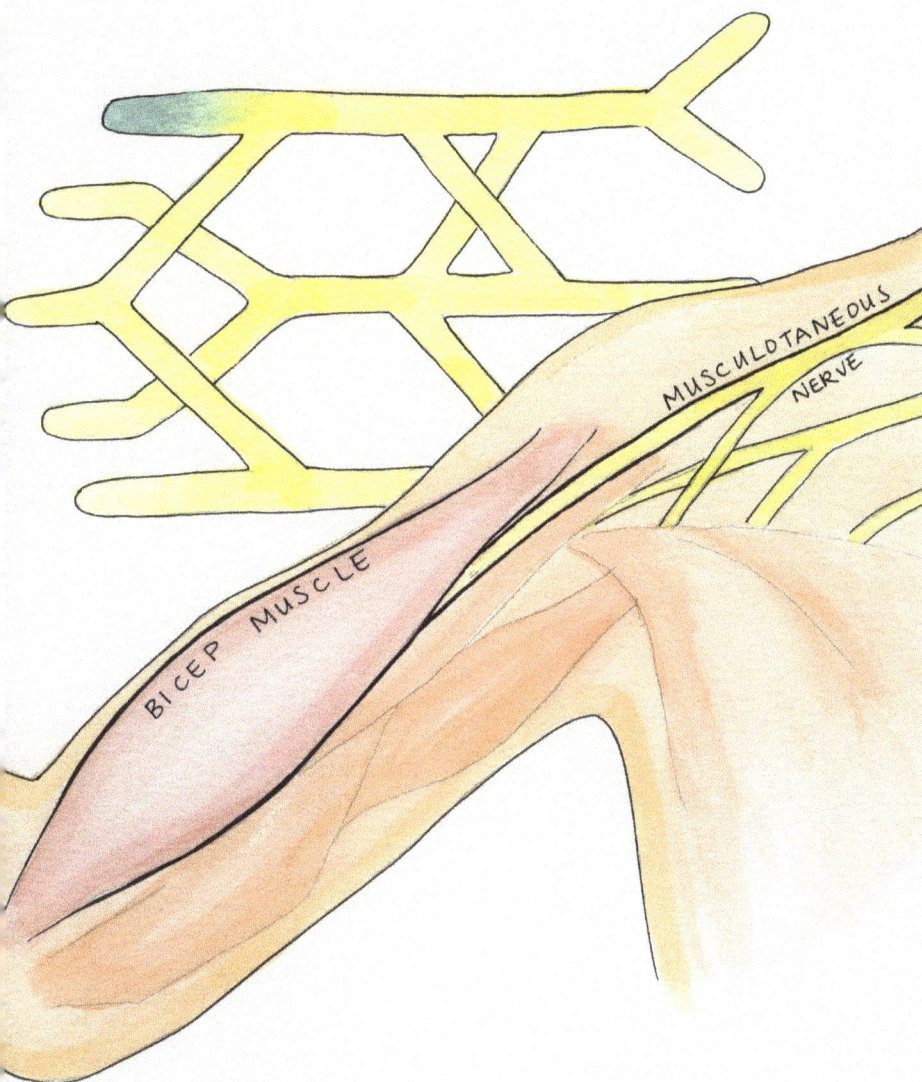

BICEP MUSCLE

MUSCULOCUTANEOUS NERVE

M IS FOR MUSCULOCUTANEOUS NERVE. THE MUSCULOCUTANEOUS NERVE IS THE BRANCH OF THE BRACHIAL PLEXUS THAT INNERVATES THE BICEPS MUSCLE.

N IS FOR NERVE GRAFT. NERVE GRAFT REPAIR IS A SURGICAL PROCEDURE WHERE A NERVE FROM ANOTHER PORTION OF THE BODY IS USED TO REPLACE THE NERVE THAT IS NOT FUNCTIONING PROPERLY. THE PURPOSE IS TO SERVE ONLY AS A CONDUIT THROUGH WHICH A RE-GROWING NERVE MUST PASS. USUALLY THE SURAL NERVE FROM THE LEG IS USED AS A NERVE GRAFT.

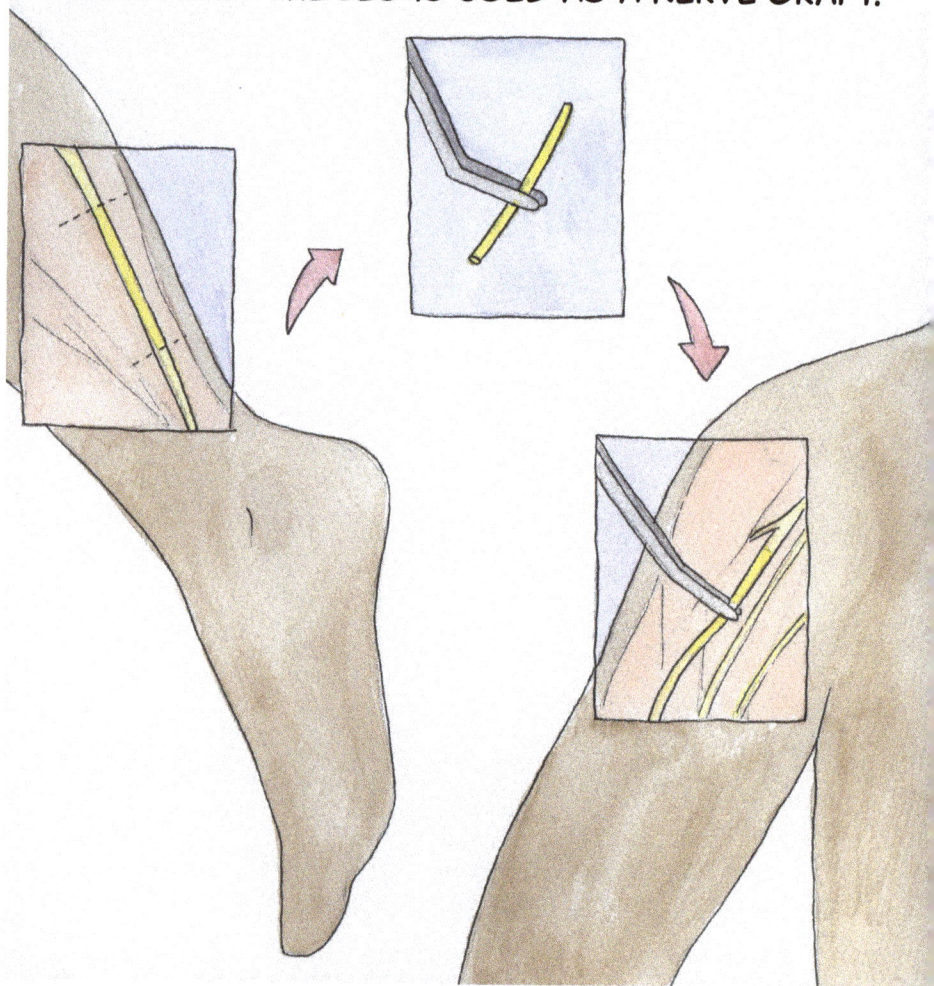

N IS FOR NEURAPRAXIA. NEURAPRAXIA IS A BLOCKAGE OF THE OUTER LAYERS OR MEMBRANES OF NERVES AS A RESULT OF STRETCH OR COMPRESSION. SURGERY IS GENERALLY NOT REQUIRED, AND RECOVERY USUALLY OCCURS IN 4-6 WEEKS.

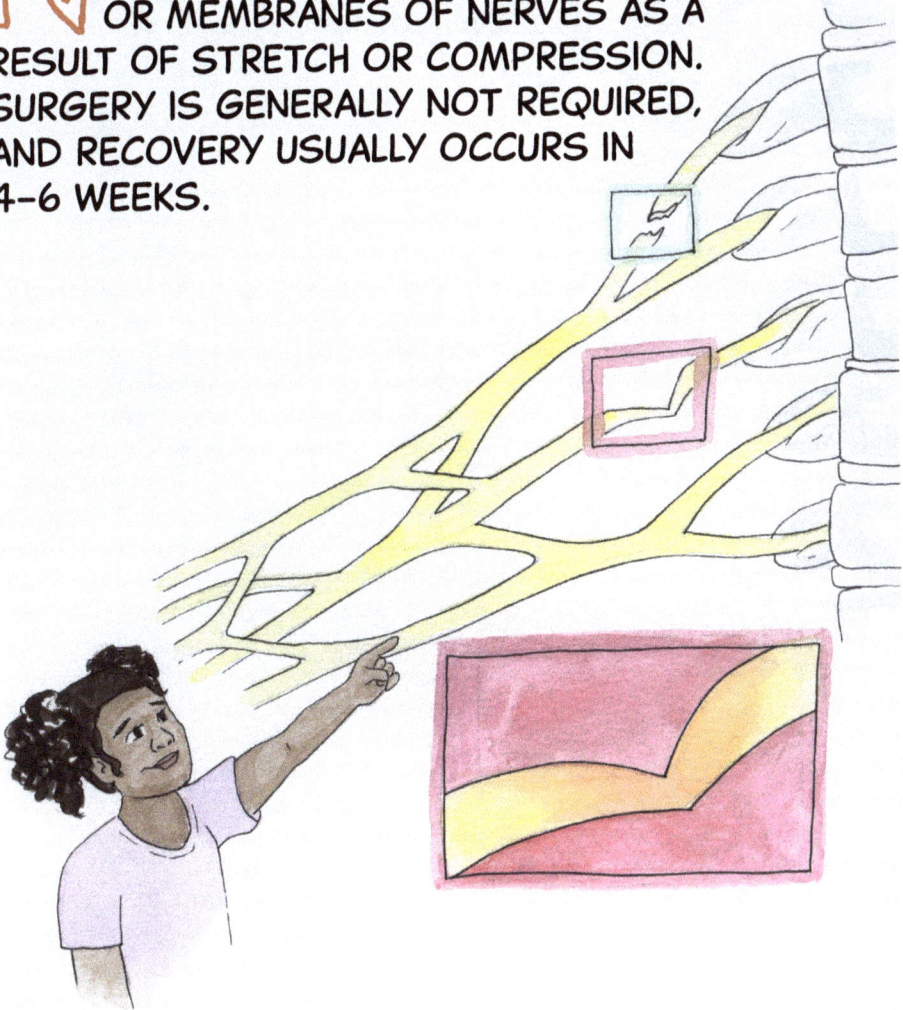

N IS FOR NEUROMA. NEUROMA IS A COMBINATION OF A DISORGANIZED MASS OF RE-GROWING NERVES AND SCAR TISSUE THAT FORMS WHEN THE NERVES OF THE BRACHIAL PLEXUS HAVE BEEN STRETCHED OR TORN.

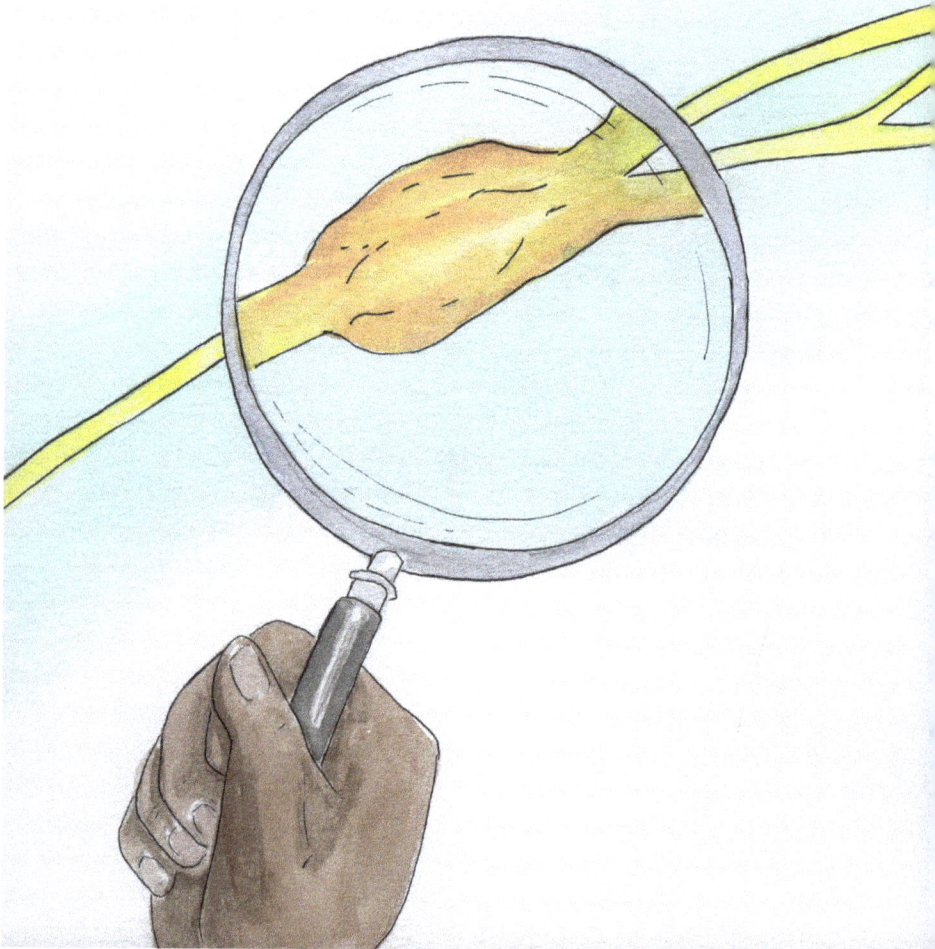

ABCs OF THE BRACHIAL PLEXUS

N IS FOR NEUROTIZATION. NEUROTIZATION, OR NERVE TRANSFER, IS A SURGICAL PROCEDURE WHERE PART OF A HEALTHY NERVE IS RE-ROUTED TO A NERVE THAT IS NOT FUNCTIONING PROPERLY, OR DIRECTLY INTO A MUSCLE THAT IS WEAK.

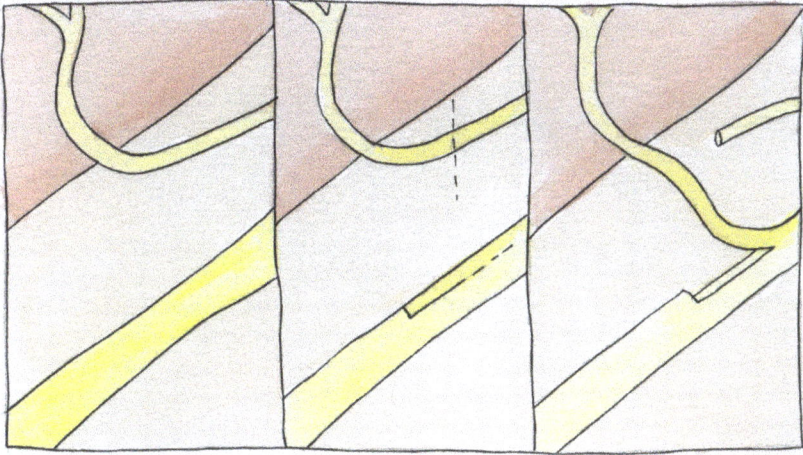

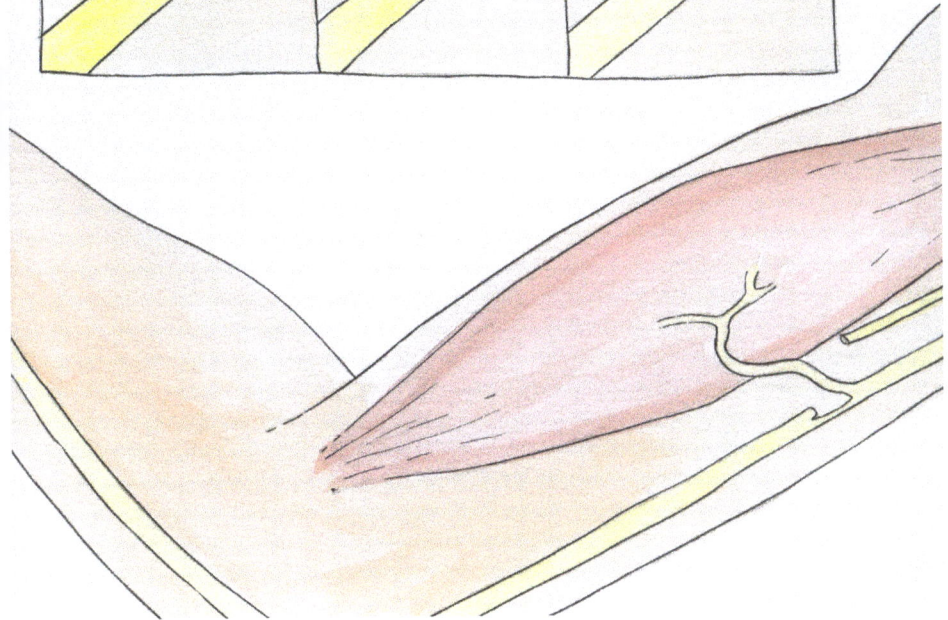

ABCs OF THE BRACHIAL PLEXUS

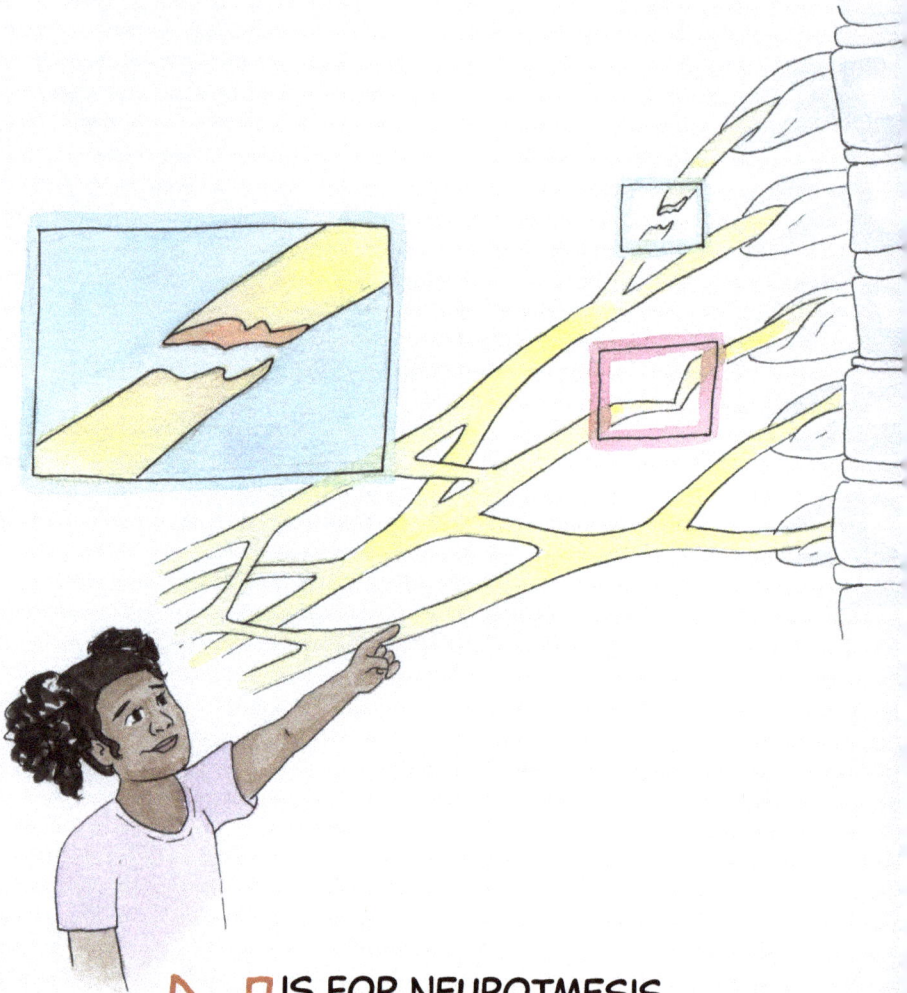

N IS FOR NEUROTMESIS.
NEUROTMESIS MEANS COMPLETE
SEPARATION OF ALL LAYERS OF A
NERVE. SURGICAL REPAIR OF THE NERVE
IS NECESSARY TO RECOVER FUNCTION.

ABCs OF THE BRACHIAL PLEXUS

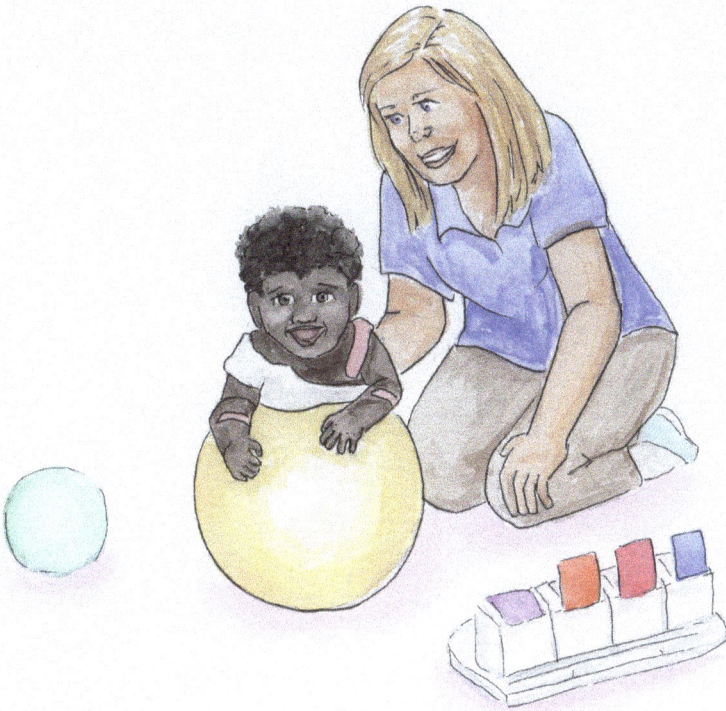

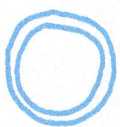

O IS FOR OCCUPATIONAL OR PHYSICAL THERAPY. OCCUPATIONAL OR PHYSICAL THERAPY IS OFTEN RECOMMENDED TO ASSIST A CHILD WITH A NEONATAL BRACHIAL PLEXUS PALSY TO STRENGTHEN THE WEAK ARM AND TO ACHIEVE INDEPENDENCE WITH ACTIVITIES OF DAILY LIVING, OR TO HELP DEVELOP LARGE AND SMALL MUSCLE MOTOR SKILLS.

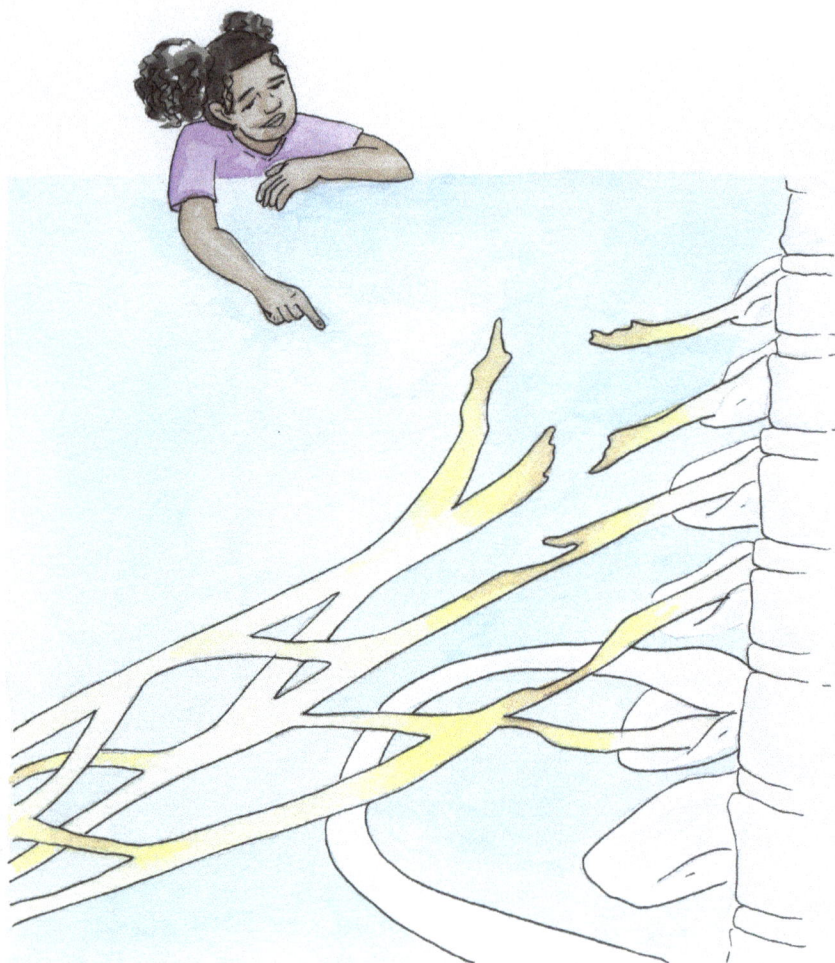

P IS FOR PAN-PLEXOPATHY. PAN-PLEXOPATHY OCCURS WITH A STRETCH, RUPTURE, OR AVULSION TO THE NERVES OF THE ENTIRE BRACHIAL PLEXUS. THIS IS THE MOST EXTENSIVE FORM OF NEONATAL BRACHIAL PLEXUS PALSY.

ABCs OF THE BRACHIAL PLEXUS

P IS FOR PHRENIC NERVE. THE PHRENIC NERVE CONTROLS THE DIAPHRAGM. THE DIAPHRAGM IS A MUSCLE THAT SEPARATES THE CHEST FROM THE ABDOMEN AND ASSISTS WITH BREATHING.

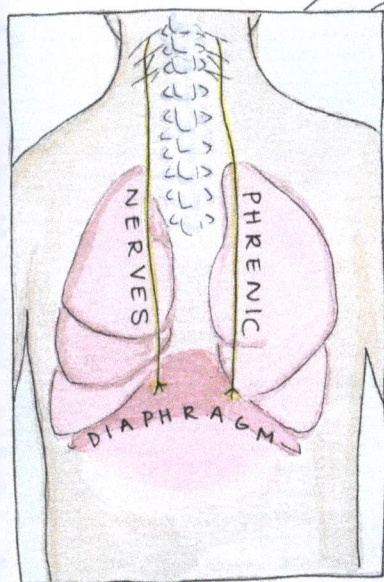

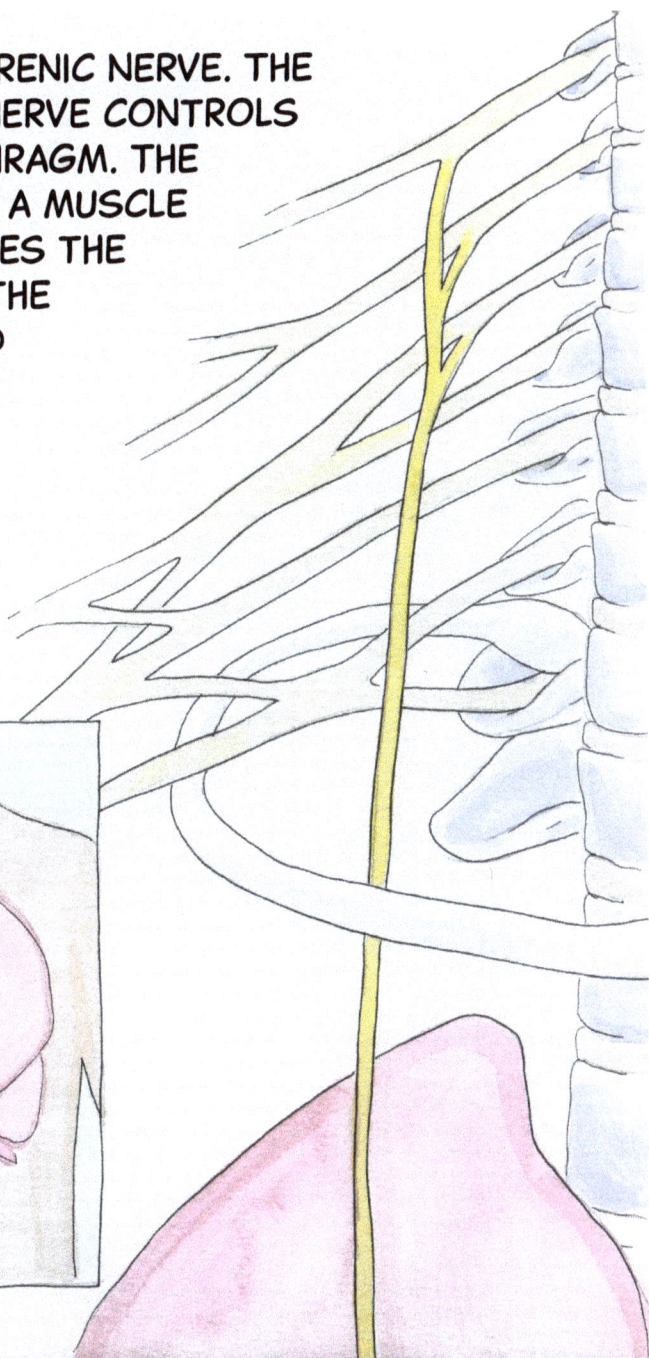

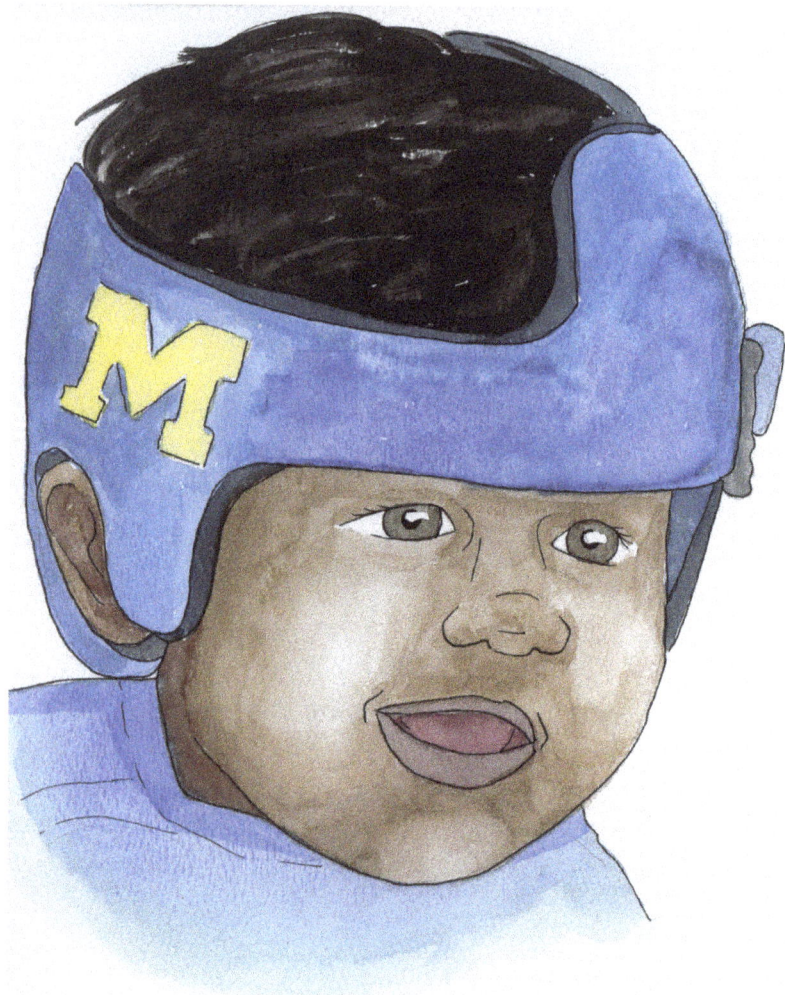

P IS FOR PLAGIOCEPHALY. PLAGIOCEPHALY MEANS THE HEAD IS MISSHAPEN. FLATTENING OF THE BACK OF THE HEAD COMMONLY RESULTS FROM TORTICOLLIS. ONE POSSIBLE TREATMENT FOR PLAGIOCEPHALY IS HELMET THERAPY, WHICH CAN HELP CORRECT THE SHAPE OF THE HEAD.

ABCs OF THE BRACHIAL PLEXUS

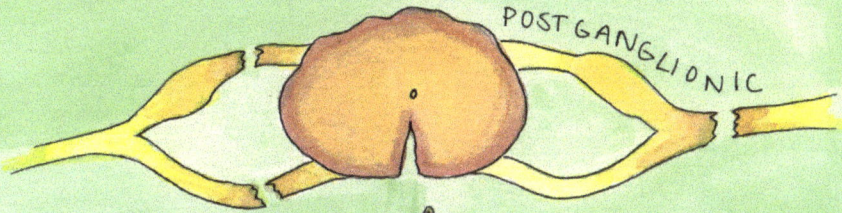

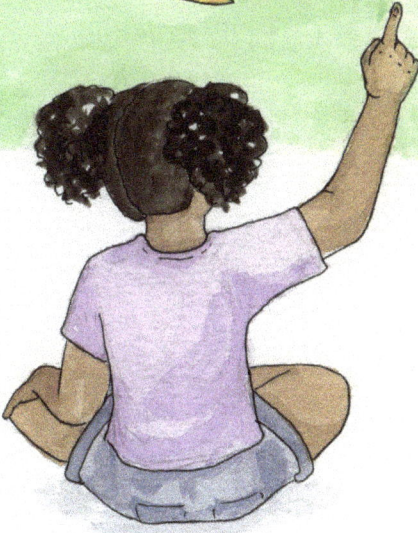

P IS FOR POST-GANGLIONIC. POST-GANGLIONIC INJURY OR RUPTURE OCCURS WHEN THE NERVE OUTSIDE OF THE SPINAL CANAL IS DISRUPTED. SURGICAL INTERVENTION MAY BE INDICATED. RECOVERY WITHOUT SURGERY IS UNPREDICTABLE.

ABCs OF THE BRACHIAL PLEXUS

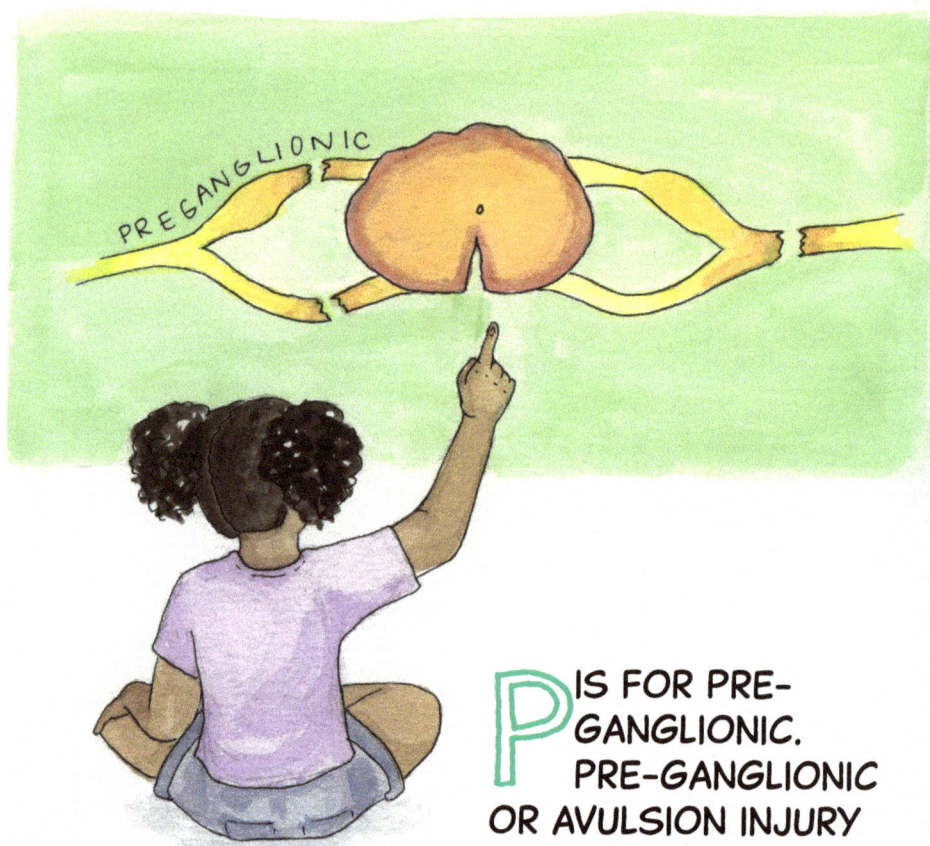

PREGANGLIONIC

P IS FOR PRE-GANGLIONIC. PRE-GANGLIONIC OR AVULSION INJURY OCCURS WHEN THE NERVE IS PULLED AWAY FROM THE SPINAL CORD AND IS THE MOST SEVERE FORM OF NERVE TRAUMA. SPONTANEOUS RECOVERY OF MUSCLE CONTROL DOES NOT OCCUR. A HORNER'S SIGN IS ASSOCIATED WITH AVULSION OF THE T1 NERVE. WITHOUT SURGICAL INTERVENTION, THE PROGNOSIS FOR RETURN OF MUSCLE CONTROL IS POOR.

ABCs OF THE BRACHIAL PLEXUS

NEUTRAL

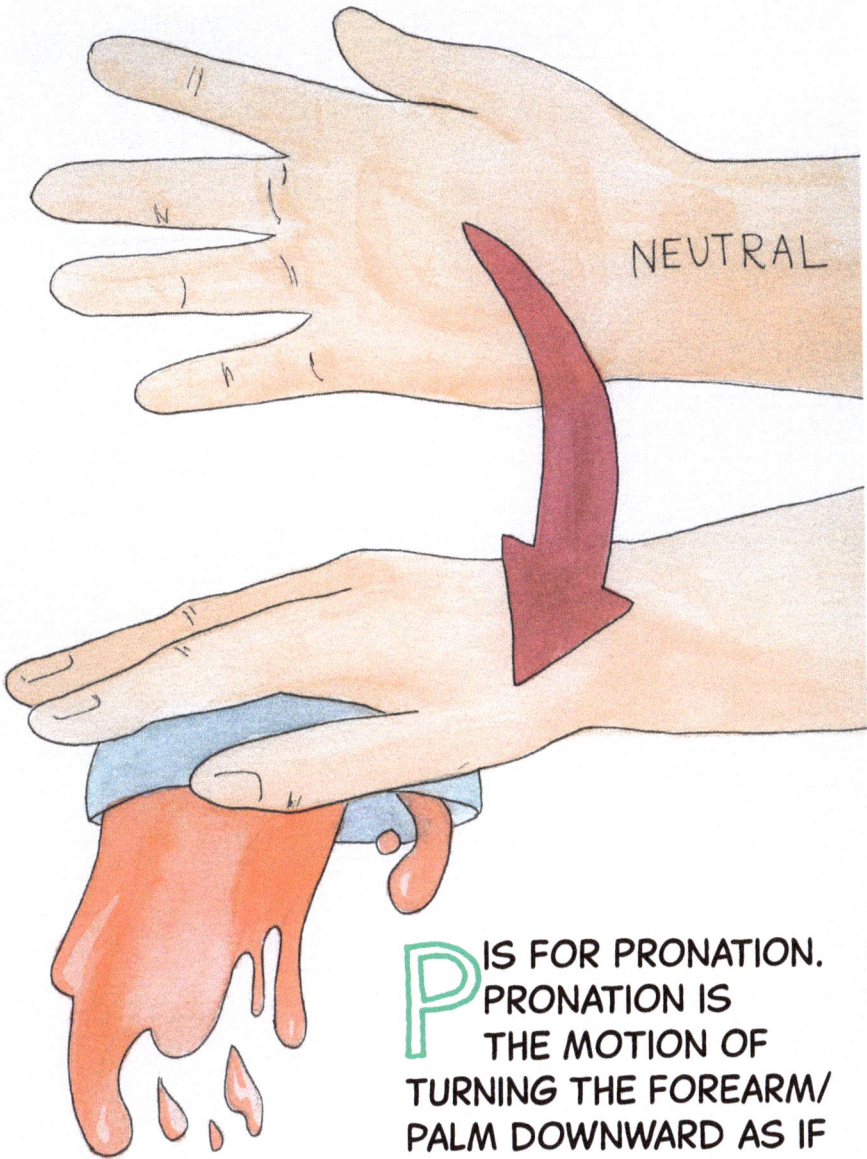

P IS FOR PRONATION.
PRONATION IS
THE MOTION OF
TURNING THE FOREARM/
PALM DOWNWARD AS IF
POURING SOUP OUT OF
A BOWL.

Q IS FOR QUALITY OF LIFE. QUALITY OF LIFE IS SOMETHING THAT ALL CHILDREN WITH NEONATAL BRACHIAL PLEXUS PALSY WILL HAVE WHEN PROVIDED THE APPROPRIATE RESOURCES AND A POSITIVE ATTITUDE.

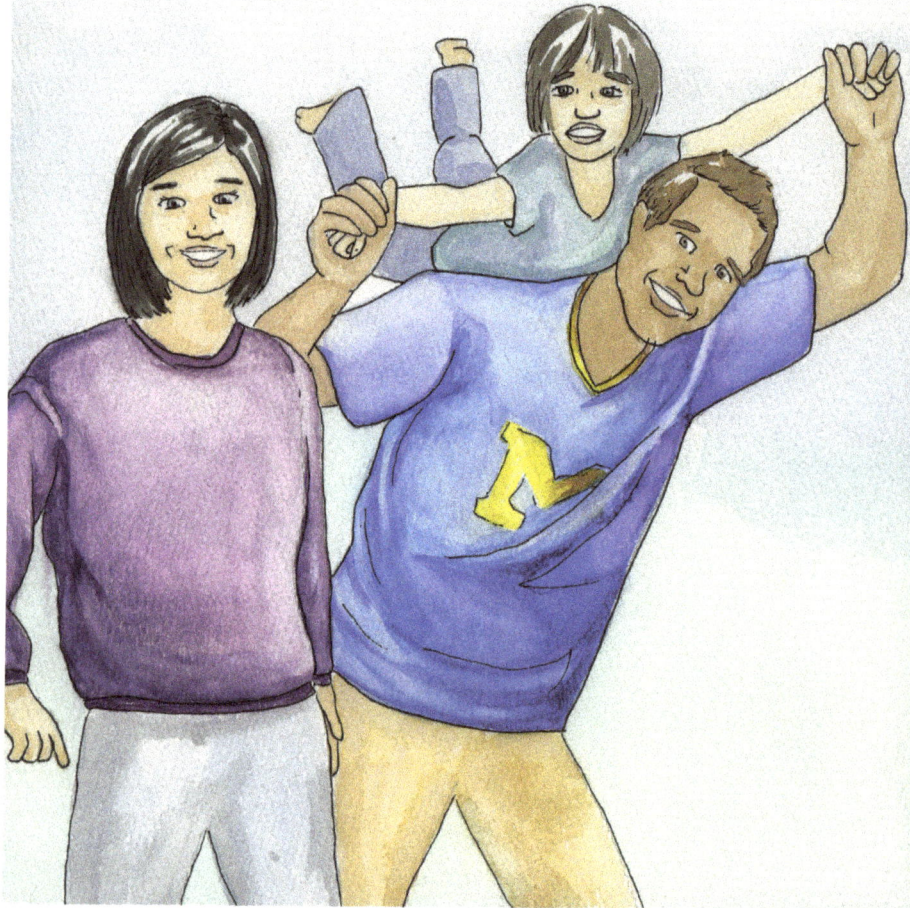

ABCs OF THE BRACHIAL PLEXUS

R IS FOR RADIAL. THE RADIAL NERVE IS THE BRANCH OF THE BRACHIAL PLEXUS THAT ALLOWS EXTENSION OF THE ELBOW, WRIST, AND FINGERS.

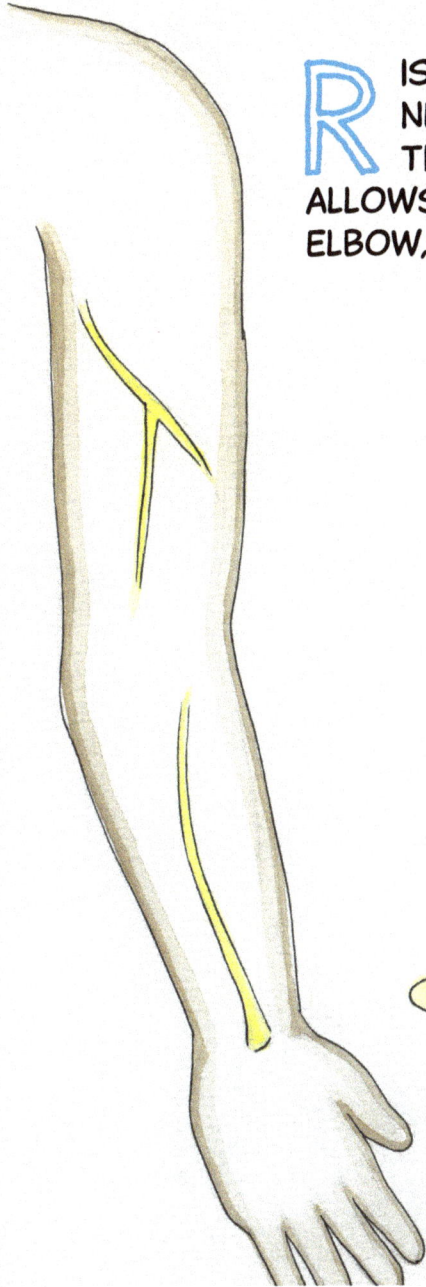

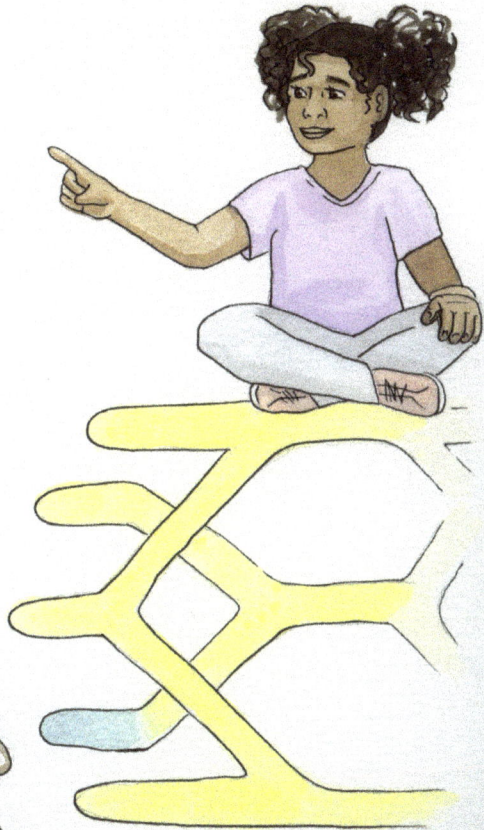

ABCs OF THE BRACHIAL PLEXUS

R IS FOR RANGE OF MOTION. RANGES OF MOTION EXERCISES ARE AN IMPORTANT PART OF CARE FOR A BABY WITH NEONATAL BRACHIAL PLEXUS PALSY. EXERCISES ARE OFTEN RECOMMENDED WITH EVERY DIAPER CHANGE DURING THE DAY. WITHOUT A FULL RANGE OF MOTION, LIMITATIONS IN ACTIVE MOVEMENT AND JOINT CONTRACTURE CAN OCCUR.

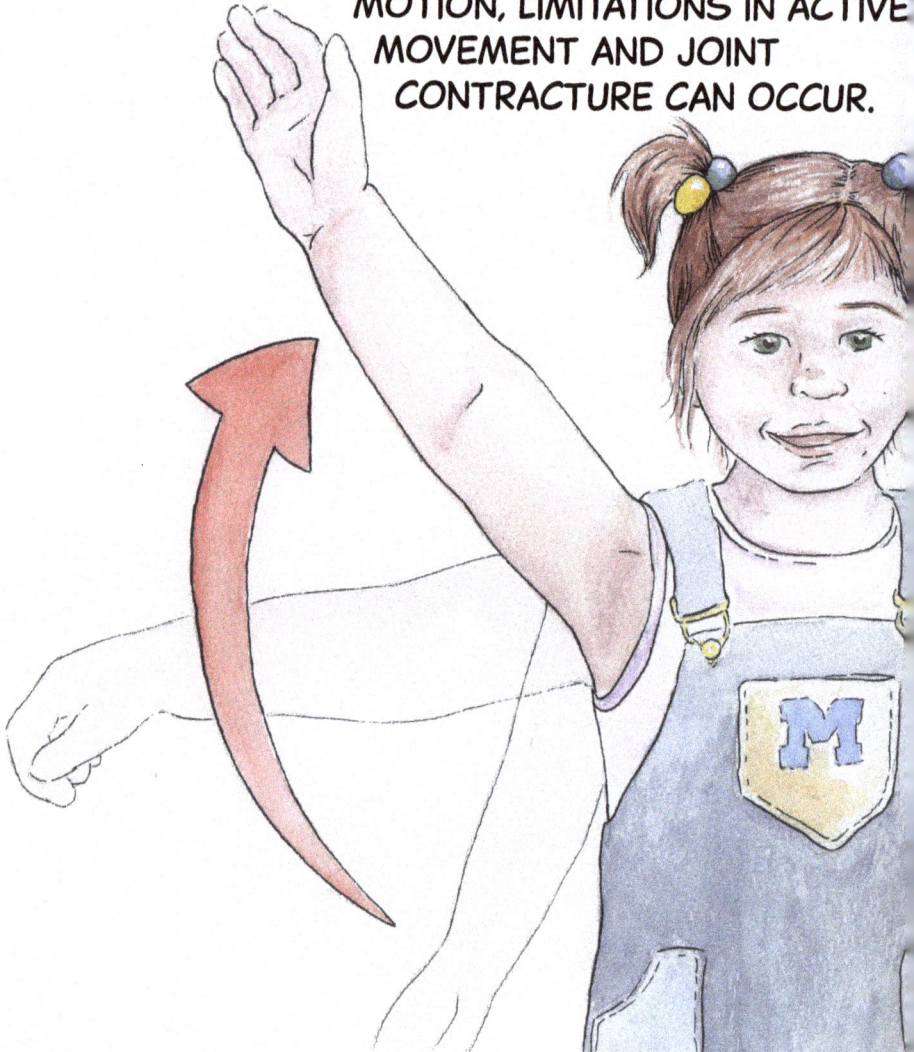

R

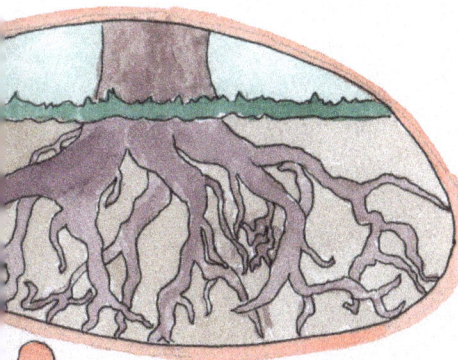

IS FOR ROOTS. ROOTS ARE THE PORTION OF THE BRACHIAL PLEXUS NERVES THAT ORIGINATE FROM THE SPINAL CORD. THERE ARE 5 ROOTS IN THE BRACHIAL PLEXUS: C5, C6, C7, C8, AND T1.

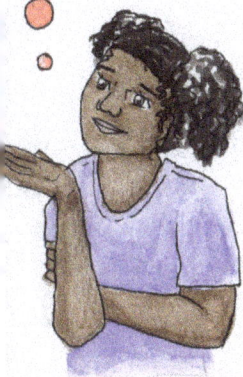

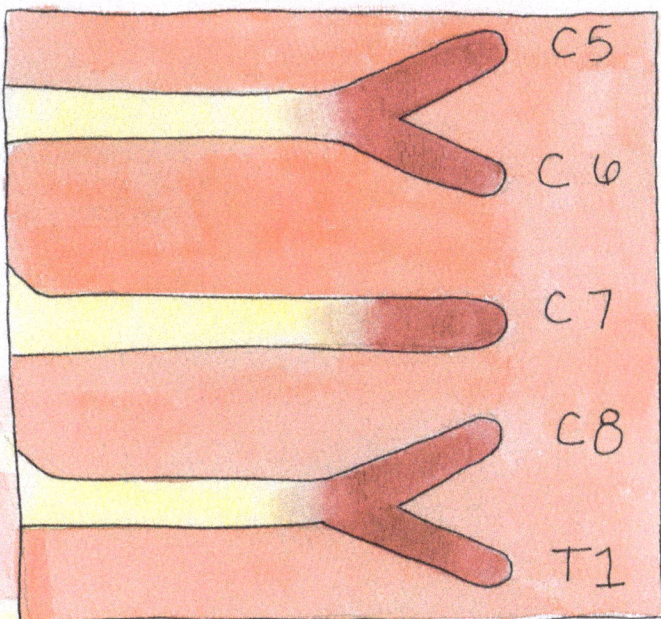

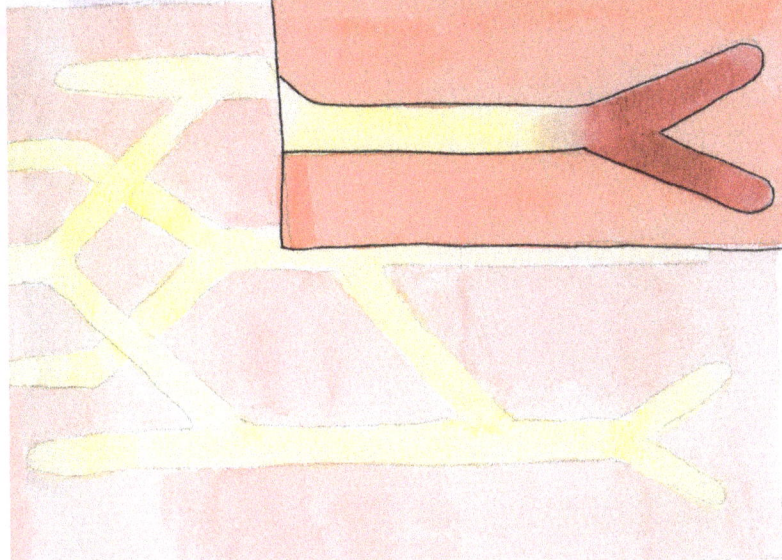

C5

C 6

C 7

C8

T1

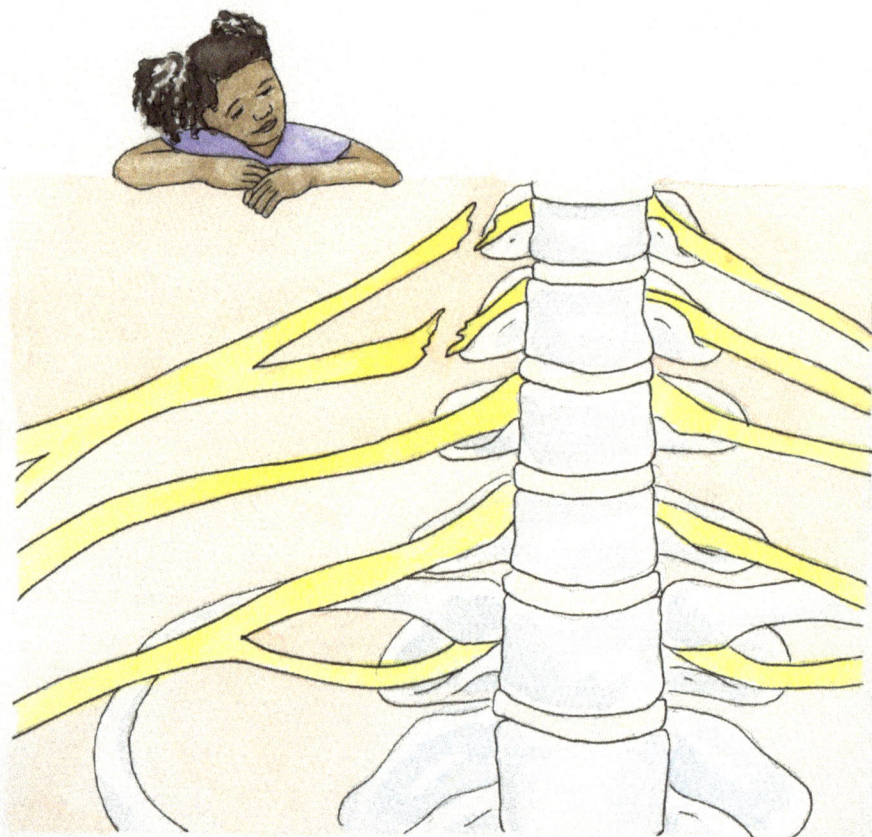

R IS FOR RUPTURE. RUPTURE MEANS
A NERVE OF THE BRACHIAL PLEXUS
HAS BEEN TORN, BUT THE NERVE IS
STILL CONNECTED TO THE SPINAL CORD.

ABCs OF THE BRACHIAL PLEXUS

S IS FOR SENSATION. SENSATION, OR THE ABILITY OF THE ARM TO FEEL, CAN BE AFFECTED BY A STRETCH TO THE BRACHIAL PLEXUS. LOSS OF SENSATION CAN BE TEMPORARY OR LONG-LASTING. WHEN SENSATION RETURNS TO THE BRACHIAL PLEXUS, SOME CHILDREN WHO CANNOT EXPRESS DISCOMFORT WILL TEND TO BITE OR SCRATCH AT HIS/HER ARM AND/OR FINGERS.

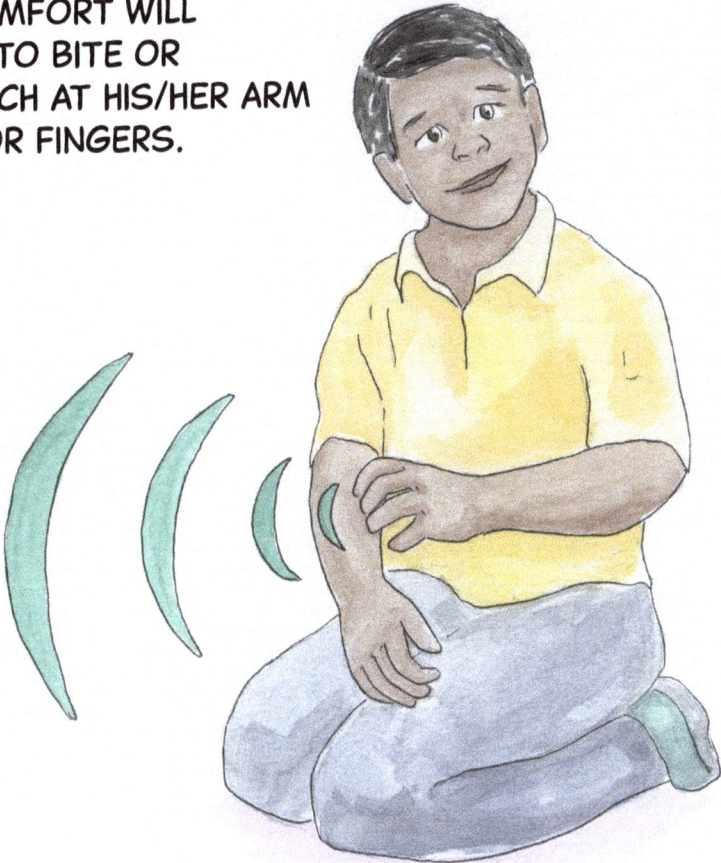

S IS FOR SHOULDER DYSTOCIA. SHOULDER DYSTOCIA OCCURS WHEN THE SHOULDER OF THE BABY IS LODGED AGAINST THE MOTHER'S PELVIC BONE (SOMETIMES THE TAIL BONE) DURING DELIVERY.

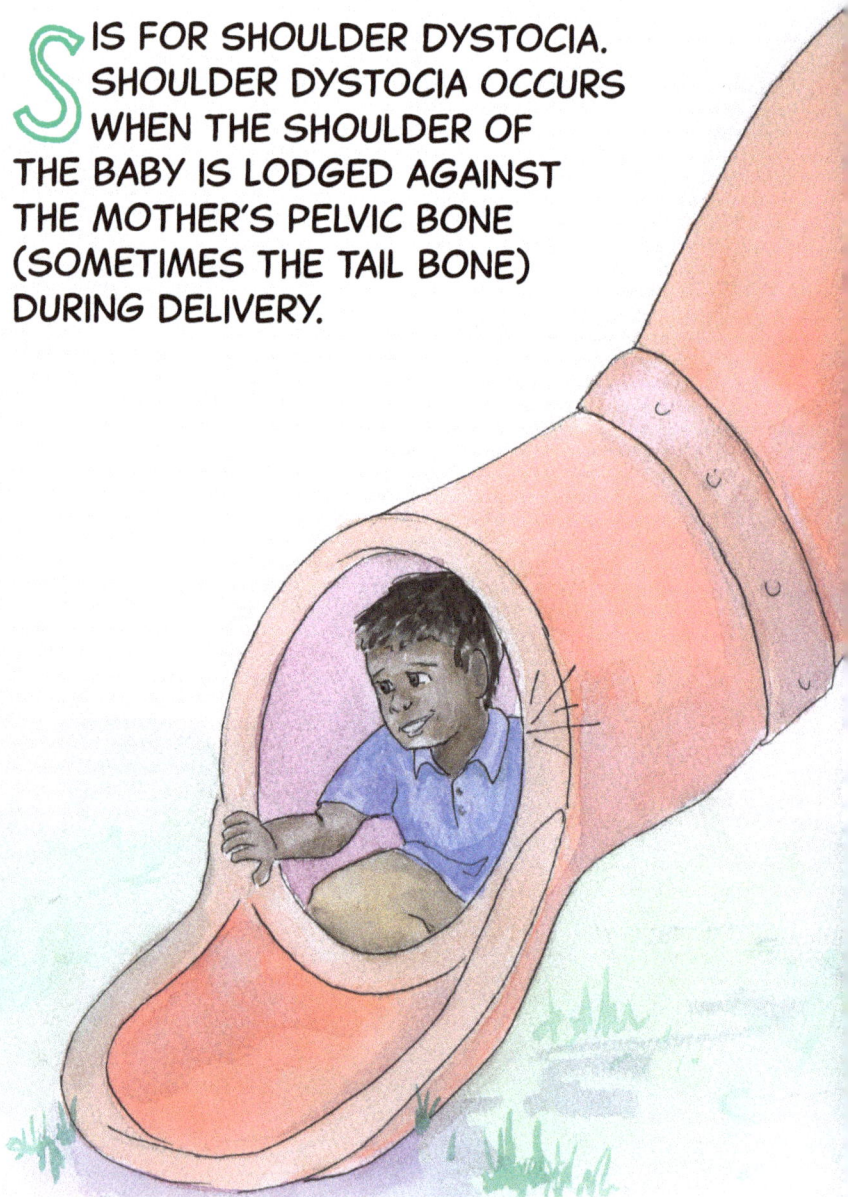

S IS FOR SPLINTS. SPLINTS MAY NEED TO BE WORN WHILE THE WEAK ARM IS RECOVERING.

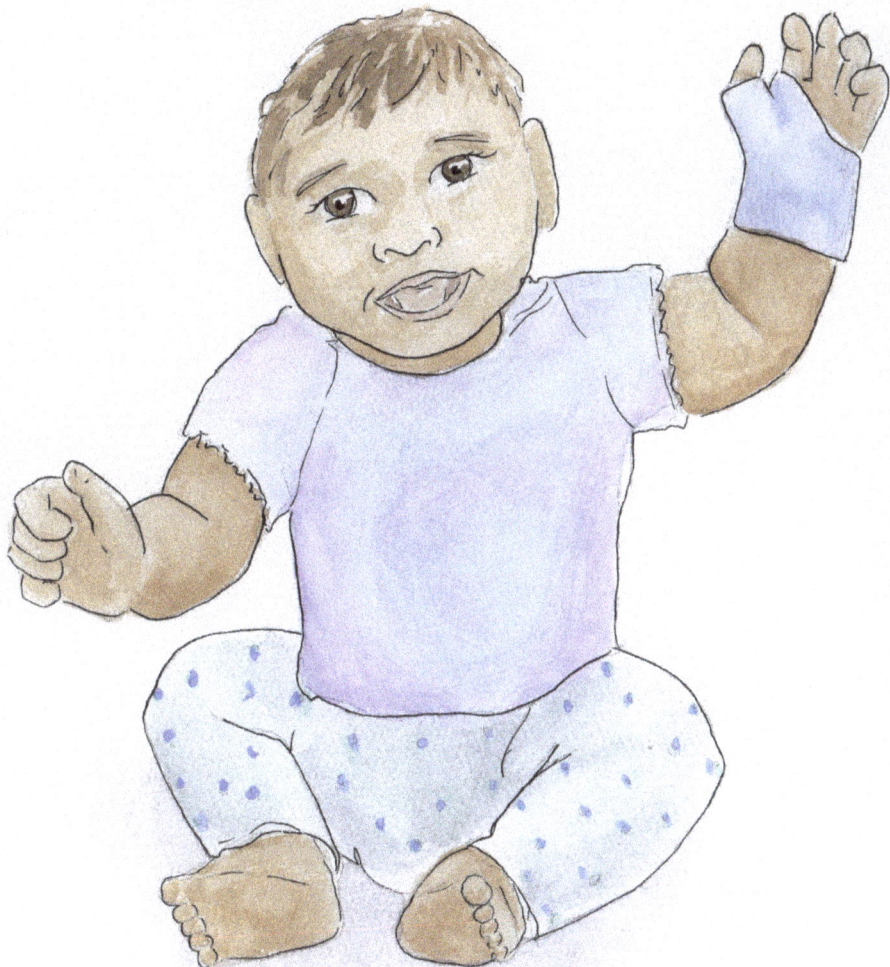

ABCs OF THE BRACHIAL PLEXUS

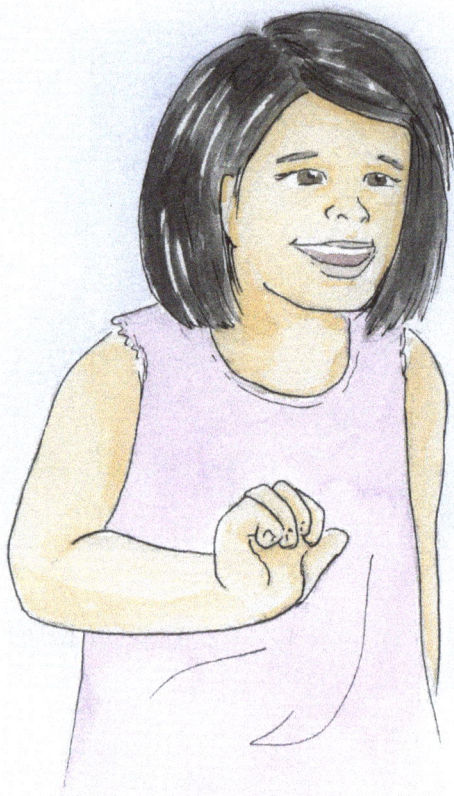

S IS FOR STEINDLER EFFECT. STEINDLER EFFECT IS THE USE OF EXTREME WRIST EXTENSION TO ASSIST WITH ELBOW FLEXION. SOME CHILDREN USE THIS MOTION TO HELP BEND THE ELBOW WHEN THE BICEPS ARE WEAK.

ABCs OF THE BRACHIAL PLEXUS

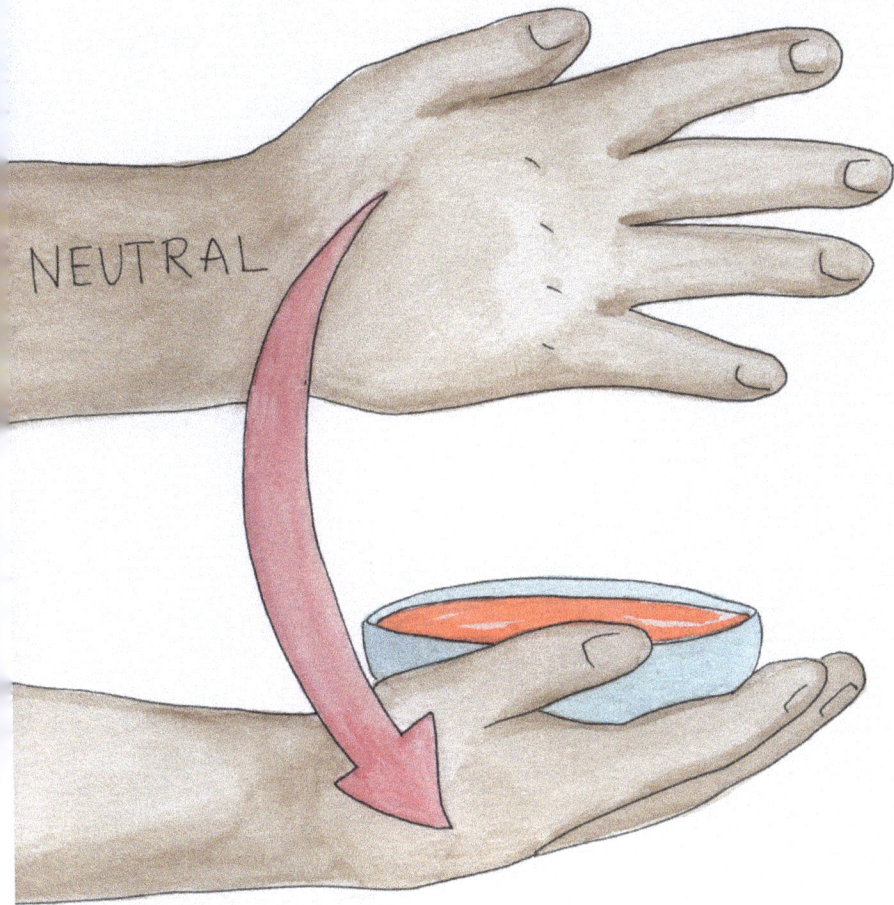

NEUTRAL

S IS FOR SUPINATION. SUPINATION IS THE MOTION OF TURNING THE FOREARM/PALM UP, AS IF YOU ARE HOLDING A BOWL OF SOUP.

S IS FOR SURAL NERVE. THE SURAL NERVE IS LOCATED IN THE BACK OF THE LEG AND SUPPLIES SENSATION TO A SMALL AREA OF THE SIDE OF THE FOOT. IT IS OFTEN REMOVED FROM THE BACK OF THE LEG AND USED TO REPAIR THE BRACHIAL PLEXUS NERVES THAT WERE STRETCHED OR TORN.

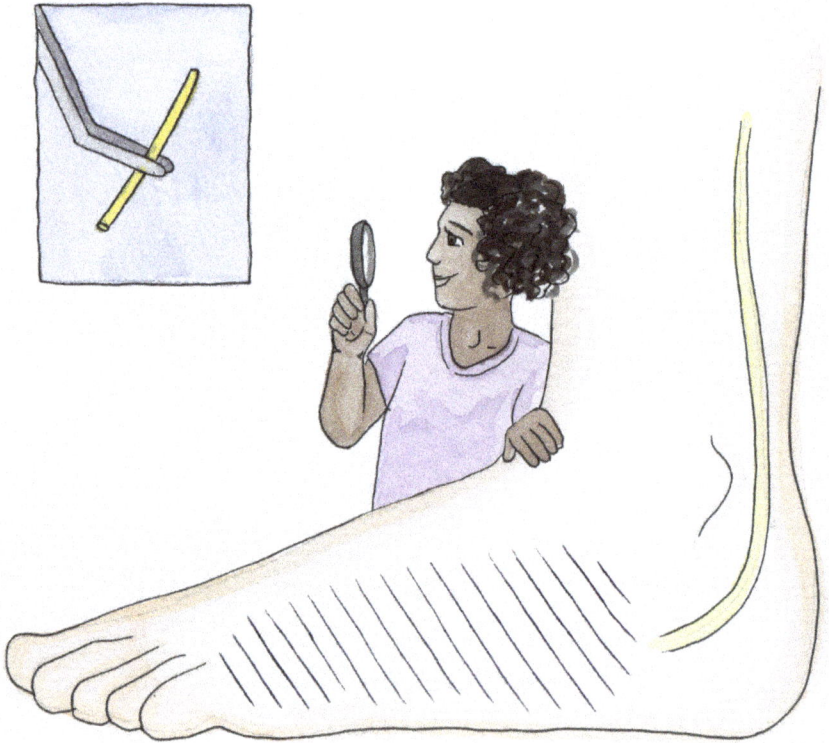

ABCs OF THE BRACHIAL PLEXUS

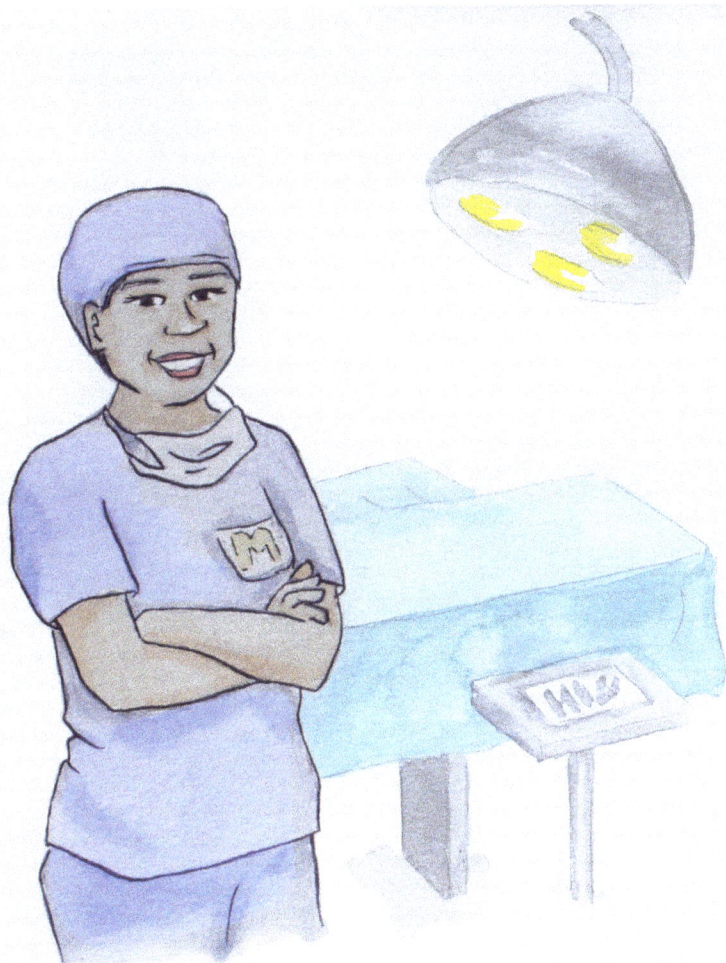

IS FOR SURGERY. SURGERY FOR NERVE
RECONSTRUCTION IS SOMETIMES NEEDED
TO RE-CONNECT, REPAIR, OR RE-ROUTE
THE NERVES TO HELP THE ARM ACQUIRE
INSTRUCTION FROM THE BRAIN TO MOVE AND
FEEL.

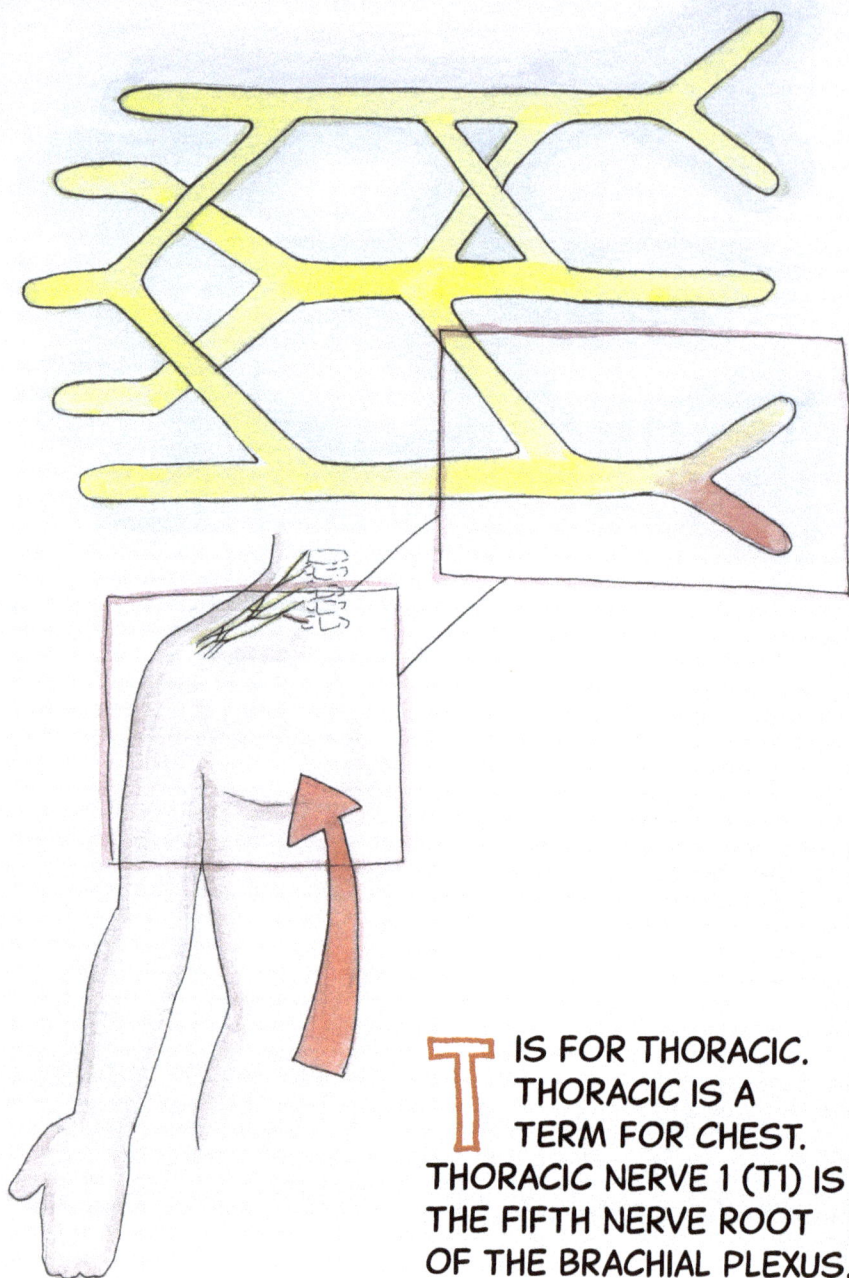

T IS FOR THORACIC.
THORACIC IS A
TERM FOR CHEST.
THORACIC NERVE 1 (T1) IS
THE FIFTH NERVE ROOT
OF THE BRACHIAL PLEXUS.

ABCs OF THE BRACHIAL PLEXUS

T IS FOR TORTICOLLIS. TORTICOLLIS CAN HAPPEN IN CHILDREN WITH OR WITHOUT NEONATAL BRACHIAL PLEXUS PALSY. TORTICOLLIS IS CHARACTERIZED BY TIGHTNESS IN THE MUSCLES OF THE NECK THAT TURN THE HEAD TO THE SIDE. TREATMENT INCLUDES NECK EXERCISES ALONG WITH BELLY TIME. SEVERE OR PROLONGED CASES OF TORTICOLLIS CAN LEAD TO PLAGIOCEPHALY.

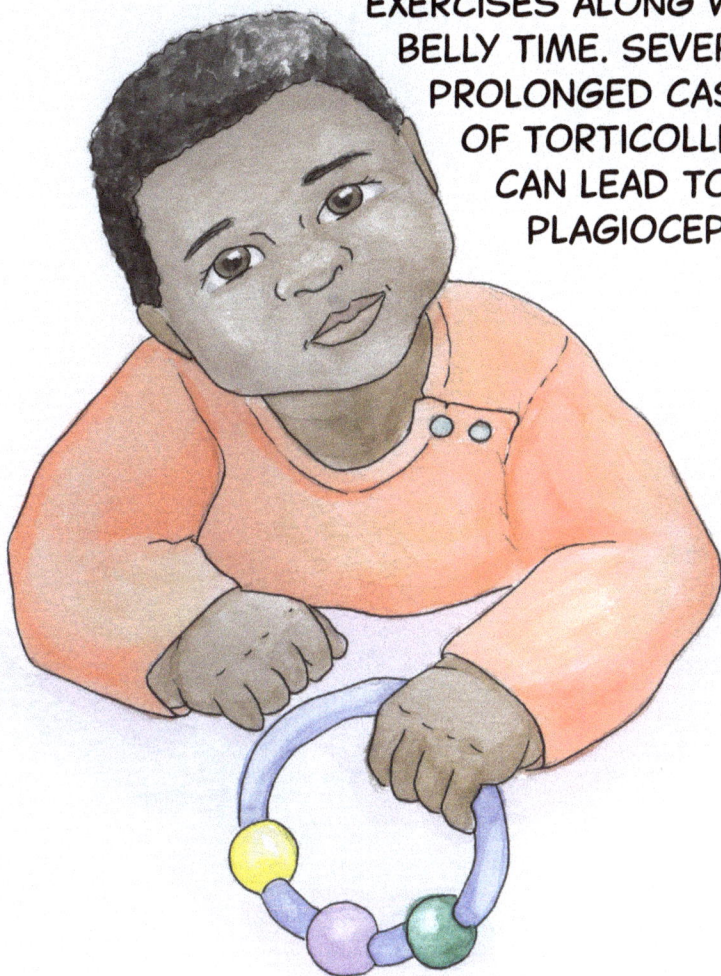

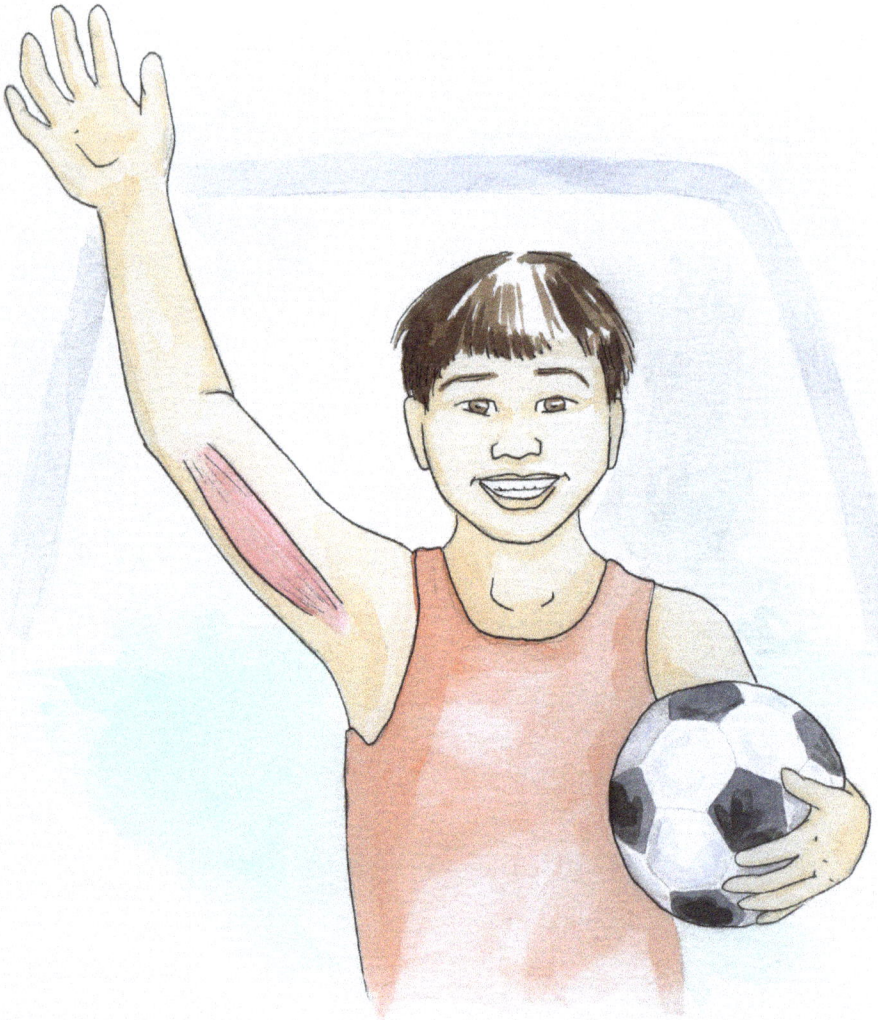

T IS FOR TRICEPS. TRICEPS IS THE MUSCLE THAT STRAIGHTENS THE ELBOW. IT IS A SIGN OF RECOVERY IF A BABY CAN STRAIGHTEN HIS/HER ELBOW AT ONE WEEK OF AGE.

ABCs OF THE BRACHIAL PLEXUS

T IS FOR TRUMPETER'S SIGN.
TRUMPETER'S SIGN DESCRIBES THE
POSITION OF THE WEAK ARM WITH
THE ELBOW ELEVATED AND LOOKS AS
IF THE CHILD IS PLAYING A TRUMPET.
THE POSTURING IS A
RESULT OF WEAKNESS
IN THE MUSCLES THAT
EXTERNALLY ROTATE
THE ARM.

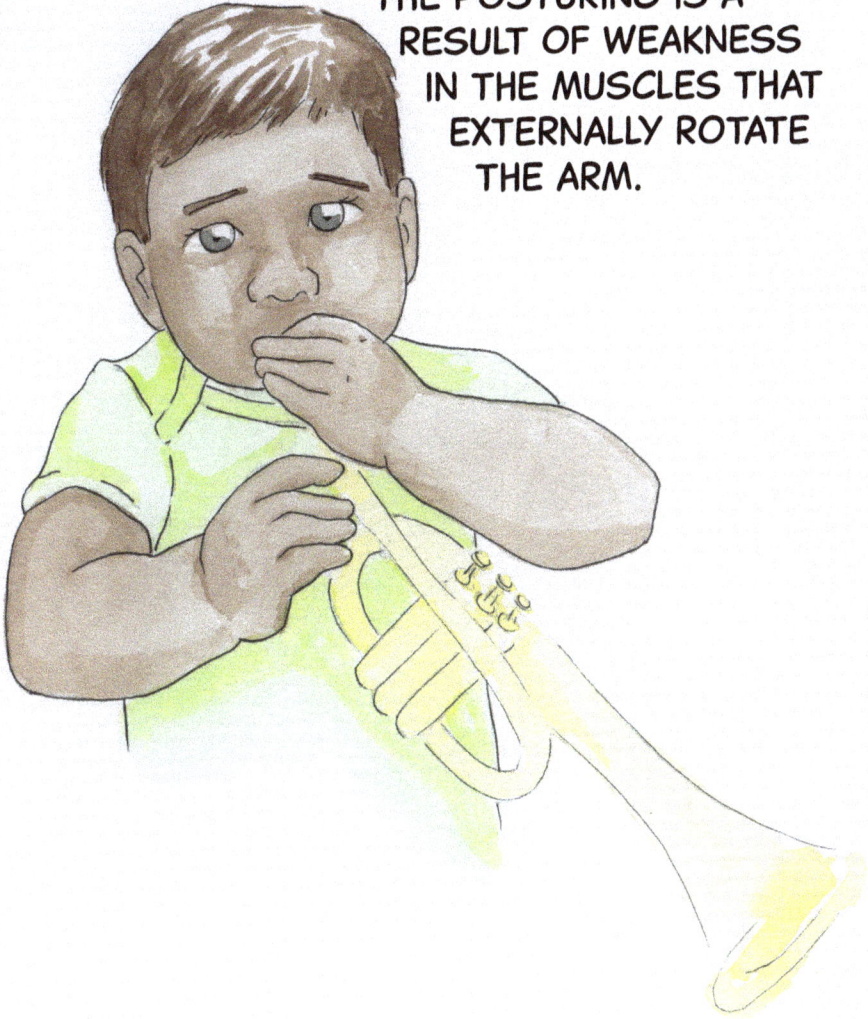

ABCs OF THE BRACHIAL PLEXUS

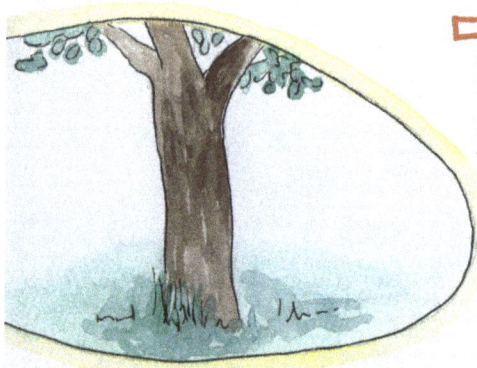

T IS FOR TRUNK. NERVE TRUNKS ARE THE SECOND PORTION OF THE BRACHIAL PLEXUS AND INCLUDE SUPERIOR (UPPER), MIDDLE, AND INFERIOR (LOWER) TRUNKS.

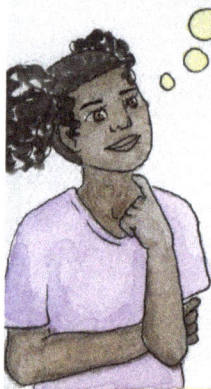

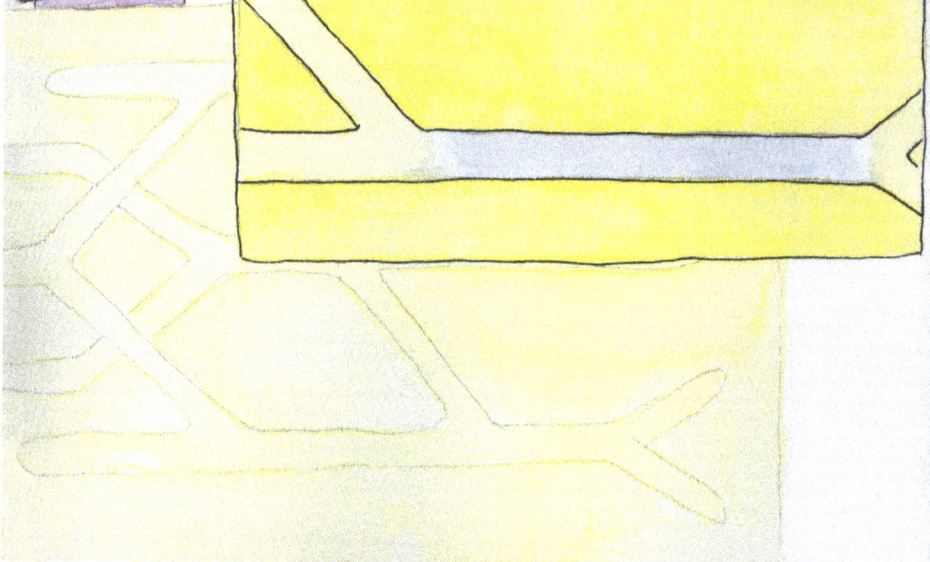

ABCs OF THE BRACHIAL PLEXUS

U IS FOR ULNAR NERVE. THE ULNAR NERVE IS THE BRANCH OF THE BRACHIAL PLEXUS THAT CONTROLS MOST OF THE MUSCLES IN THE HAND; IN PARTICULAR, SPREADING THE FINGERS APART AND BRINGING THEM TOGETHER.

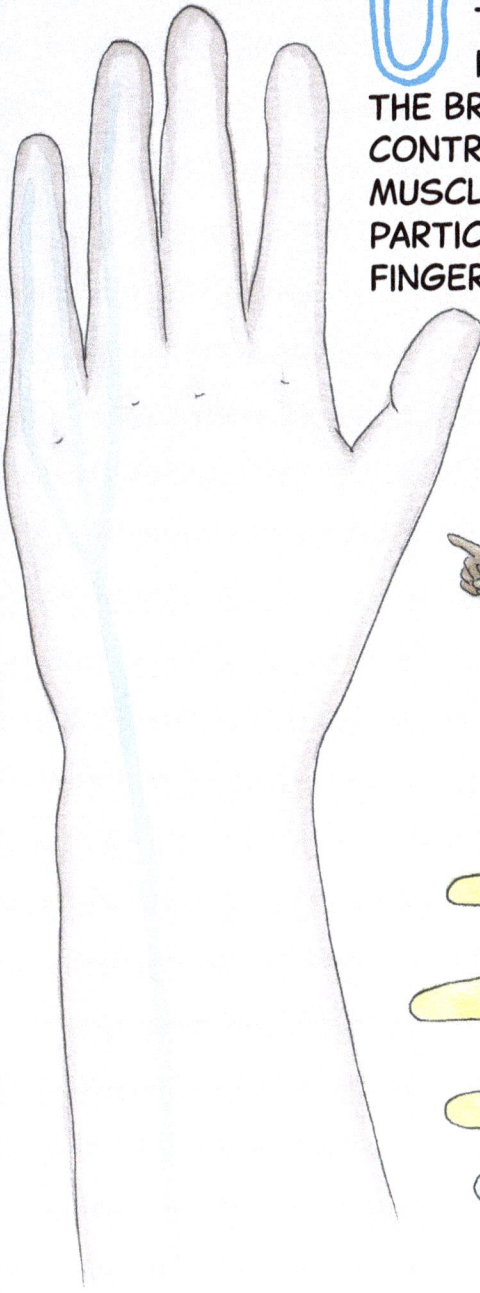

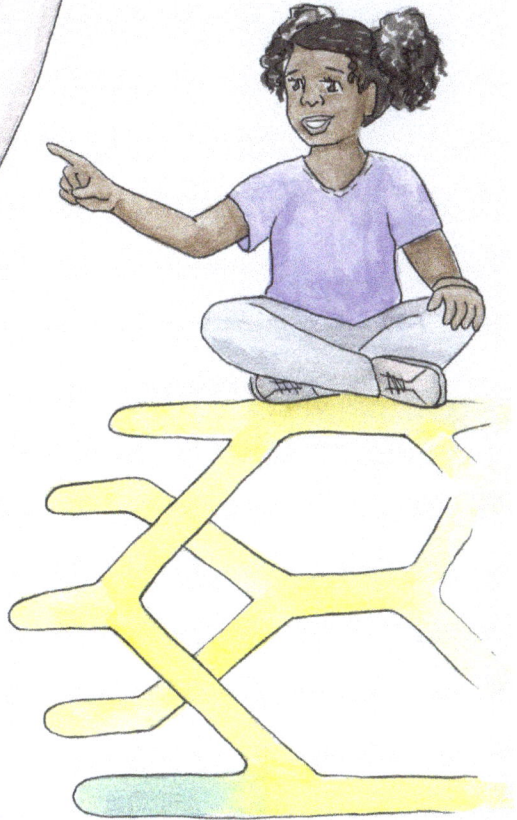

V

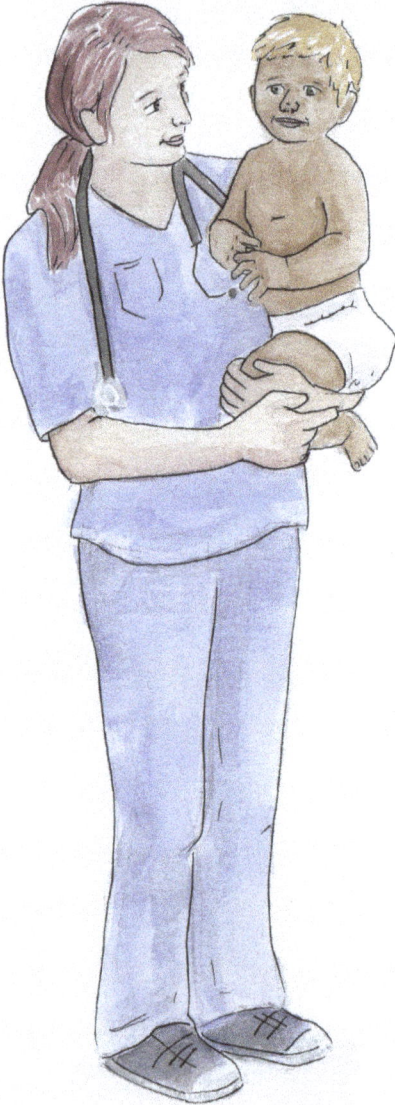

V IS FOR VISITS. VISITS TO THE SPECIALISTS MAY OCCUR EVERY 1–3 MONTHS FOR THE FIRST YEAR OF A BABY'S LIFE.

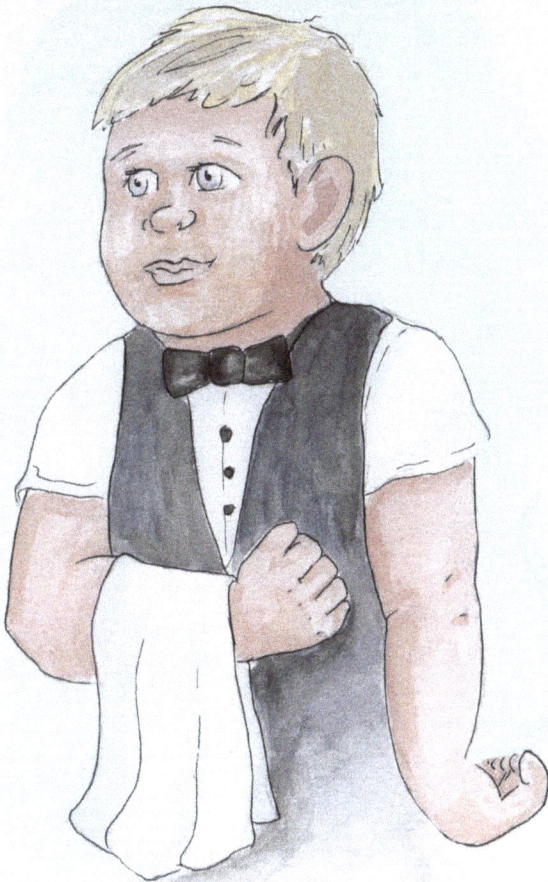

W IS FOR WAITER'S TIP. WAITER'S TIP IS THE POSTURE OF THE ARM IN CHILDREN WITH NEONATAL BRACHIAL PLEXUS PALSY THAT IS CHARACTERIZED BY SHOULDER INTERNAL ROTATION, SHOULDER ADDUCTION, ELBOW EXTENSION, FOREARM PRONATION, AND WRIST FLEXION WITH FINGERS PARTIALLY FLEXED. IT LOOKS AS THOUGH THE CHILD IS READY TO SECRETLY ACCEPT A TIP BEHIND HIS/HER BACK.

ABCs OF THE BRACHIAL PLEXUS

W IS FOR WEAKNESS. WEAKNESS IS ALSO REFERRED TO AS PARALYSIS OR PARESIS AND RESULTS FROM MUSCLE WASTING WITH OR WITHOUT NERVE INTERRUPTION.

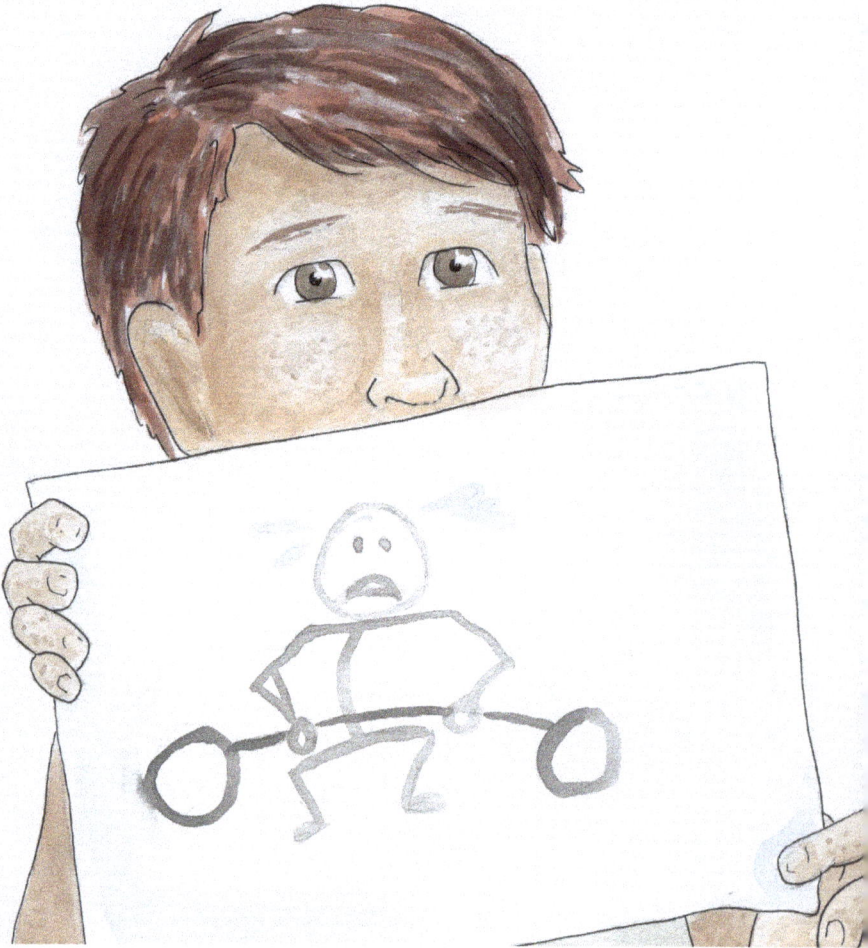

ABCs OF THE BRACHIAL PLEXUS

W

IS FOR WINGING. WINGING OF THE SCAPULA CAN OCCUR WHEN THE SHOULDER BLADE LIFTS AWAY FROM THE CHEST WALL DUE TO WEAK SHOULDER MUSCLES. SOME WINGING IS EXPECTED; SIGNIFICANT AMOUNTS OF SCAPULAR WINGING THAT INTERFERE WITH A CHILD'S ABILITY TO MOVE MAY REQUIRE THERAPEUTIC OR SURGICAL INTERVENTIONS.

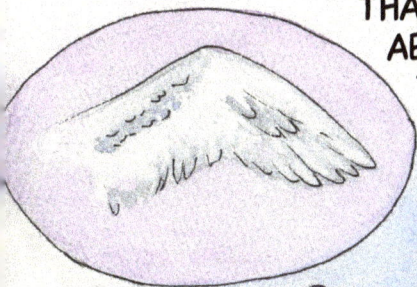

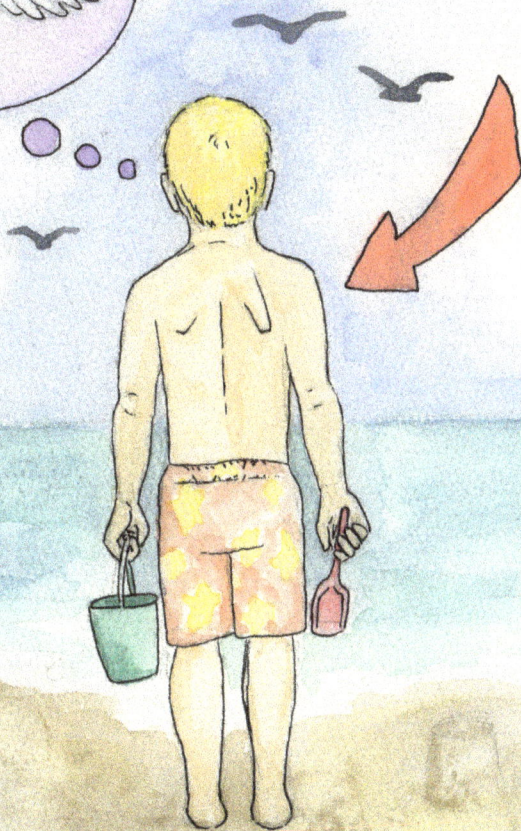

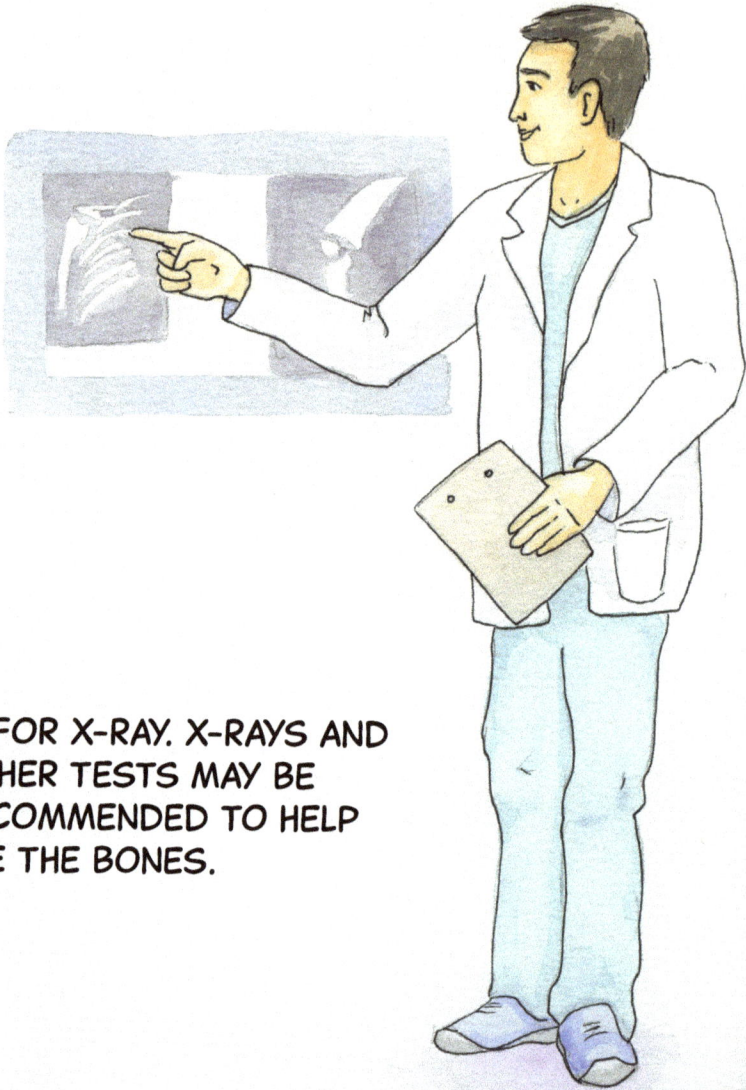

X IS FOR X-RAY. X-RAYS AND OTHER TESTS MAY BE RECOMMENDED TO HELP EVALUATE THE BONES.

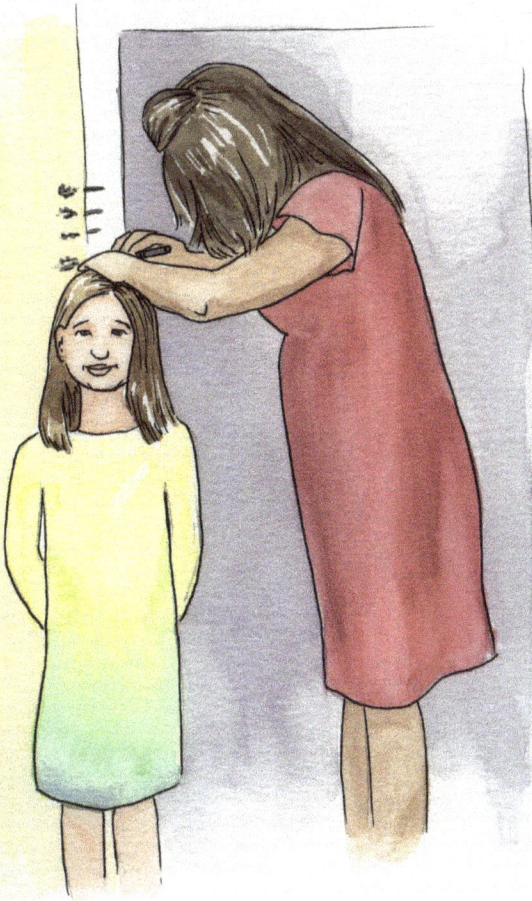

Y IS FOR YEARS. YEARS MAY BE THE AMOUNT OF TIME THAT IS NEEDED FOR THE NERVES OF THE BRACHIAL PLEXUS TO REGENERATE, WHICH USUALLY OCCURS AT A RATE OF 1 MILLIMETER PER DAY OR 1 INCH PER MONTH.

Z IS FOR ZIPPIEST. ZIPPIEST IS THE FASTEST RECOVERY THE MEDICAL PROVIDERS STRIVE TO ACHIEVE.

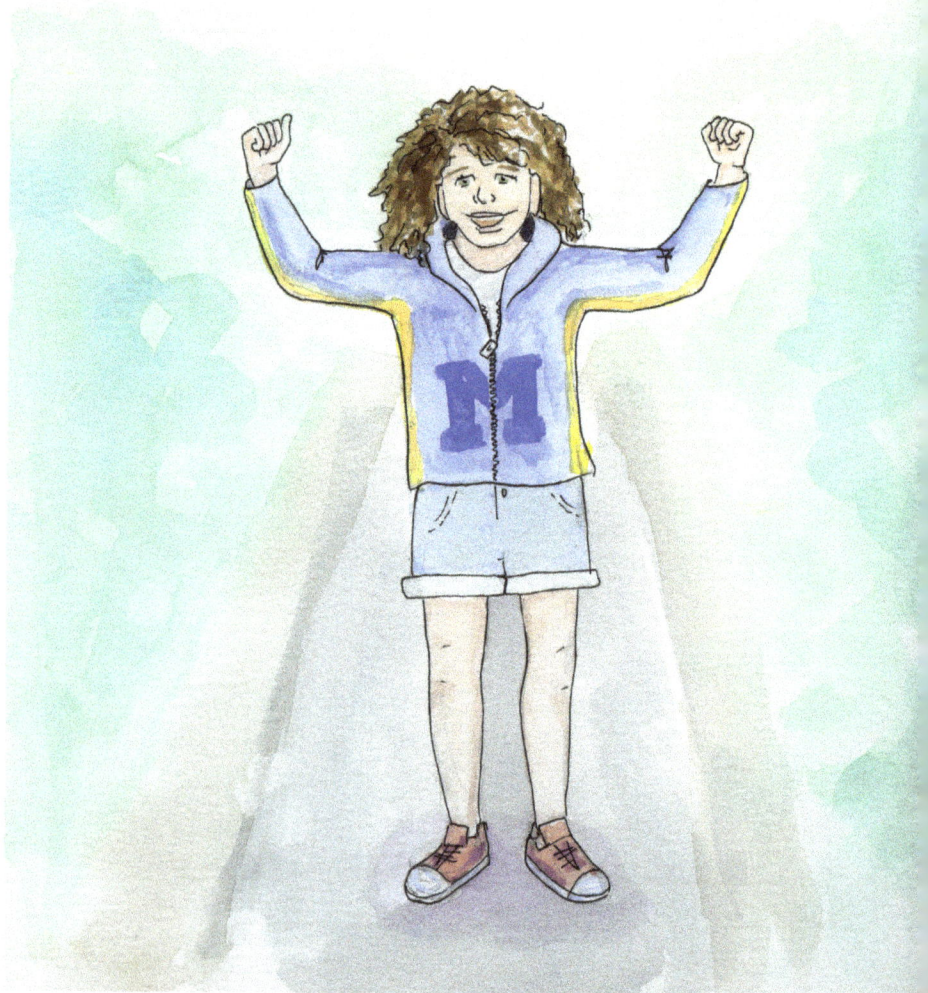

ABCs OF THE BRACHIAL PLEXUS

INDEX OF TERMS

INDEX OF TERMS

www.ingramcontent.com/pod-product-compliance
Lightning Source LLC
Chambersburg PA
CBHW042139210326
41521CB00036B/2602